Free Gift

This book includes a bonus booklet. This giveaway may be for a limited time only. All information on how you can secure your gift right now can be found at the end of this book.

Table of Contents

<u>YOUR FREE GIFT IS HERE!</u>

Book Description:

Do you smoke one cigarette after the other, and wish you could find a way to quit? This is the no-nonsense guide you need to read so that you can stop smoking forever.

Diseases, bothering other people, coughing, always feeling unhealthy; nothing good comes from smoking, and yet you can't seem to stop. It's 2019, and 'I don't know how' is just not an excuse anymore. Your health and your life are on the line. It's time to say goodbye to your addiction.

In *Stop Smoking,* I take you through a step by step process that will convince you to stop and then teach you how to make that stick. Your body is desperate to be healthy again. That is why this guide is going to be the turning point for you, the final stop on your road to being a non-smoker!

In this step by step guide you'll discover:

- Why you should quit smoking right now (not tomorrow)
- How smoking affects your body, mind and those around you
- How to prepare for the day you quit forever
- What you can expect when you quit, and how to fight back
- What your smoking triggers are, and how to change them
- How to manage the side effects after you quit (don't gain weight!)

You always knew the day would come when quitting stopped being a concept, and became a reality. This is that day. I'll teach you how to break the habit and embrace good health.

Begin the process of being healthier and happier - and breathe easy for the first time with these expert tips. Making this decision is the hard part. Then all you have to do is focus on letting go!

Become a non-smoker with this easy to use guide.
Buy it now, and stop smoking!

Introduction

So you have finally decided to kick the butt? Does the craving to light your last cigarette keep creeping in and you never manage to end the process as effectively as you had planned it in your brain? Smoking is perhaps one of the strongest addictions to overcome because your body starts to crave nicotine and the withdrawals are a little difficult to deal with.

One of the worst things about smoking is that it causes an impression of relieving stress and it feels like a release when you let go of smoke in the air. While this seems amazing and it gives you a lot of pleasure, it is one of the worst ways to abuse your body. You already know that smoking can cut short your life tremendously and can also invite a number of serious health problems. Smoking doesn't just affect you but also the people around you. There's nothing good that comes out of smoking and the sooner you understand this, the better it will be because that's going to help you quit smoking more effectively.

Giving up smoking isn't easy because the addiction is quite strong and if you've been smoking for a few years, then you need to give your body time to understand the changes that you are going to introduce. In order for you to effectively say goodbye to smoking and never turn back, you have to prepare yourself mentally and physically and this will help you take control of the situation.

If you have heard a lot of stories from people who keep telling you they attempted to quit but failed, it's because they didn't do it the right way. This guide is going to help you understand just how easy it is to say goodbye to smoking once you set your heart to do it.

This book comes with a FREE bonus chapters and gift. Instructions on how you can download this free booklet for free can be found at the bottom page of this book.

Chapter 1 - Getting Started

"The surest way not to fail is to determine to succeed." – Richard Brinsley Sheridan

6 Common Questions About Quitting Smoking

Smokers are often confused when it comes to quitting and the fright of whether or not they will manage to succeed is always there. If you want to quit smoking, you need to make sure you create a plan that doesn't fail you and you stay focused every step of the way. When it comes to quitting many questions come up in a smoker's mind but here are a few that are very common.

Why Do I Fail Every Time I Try to Quit?

It's not uncommon for smokers to try and quit smoking multiple times in their life. However, something always gets them back to smoking and they end up ditching the plan of quitting completely. Distractions are the main reason why you are not able to quit smoking and temptation comes in a close second. When you are upset about something, or you feel low, you tend to go back to smoking even if you have stayed clean for a long time. Temptation often occurs when you look at another person smoking and you suddenly feel the urge to smoke as well. Once you learn how to control both these situations, you will manage to give up smoking and succeed at it.

Should I Use Nicotine Patches to Help Me Quit?

Nicotine patches work amazing for some people, but for others, they don't work at all. It depends on how well your body adjusts to the patch. At the end of the day, it's all about figuring out what helps you stay away from smoking more effectively and what you can do to keep yourself on track and stay away from the idea of getting back to smoking.

Can I Reduce the Number of Cigarettes I Smoke Before I Quit?

While this plan seems to be great and people are often confident about lowering the number of cigarettes they smoke in the day, this plan doesn't always work. Some people believe they can narrow down their cigarettes to zero eventually. The reason this plan is flawed is that when you give yourself the leverage to smoke, you automatically increase the number of cigarettes in stressful situations instead of staying away from them. If you want to quit smoking, you have to stop it completely and face your withdrawals with a bold approach.

Can I Switch to Vape or E-Cigarettes?

While vaping and using e-cigarettes can help you quit and stop thinking about smoking for a while, the very fact that you are constantly replicating a habit that you have been trying to break keeps you wanting it more and you may want to go back to smoking just to get the feel of it. Whilst vaping and e-cigarettes can help before you quit, trying to use them once you quit smoking may not be as effective because it's a constant reminder of smoking.

Will I Feel Sick When I Quit?

Quitting is different for different people and while some of them have very little or no withdrawals, there are others who could get really irritable and cranky for the first few days. The best way for you to cope with these symptoms is to engross yourself in work or some other activity that keeps your mind busy. While withdrawal symptoms play a small part, it's your mind that keeps tricking you into wanting a cigarette because of the addiction and once you break that habit, you will manage to control your cravings more effectively.

When Should I Start?

The minute you believe you want to quit smoking, pick a date and don't look back. The more you think about it, the less motivated you will be and you will have second thoughts about whether or not you should quit smoking.

Why Quit Smoking?

We have already discussed the various health-related problems people suffer from when they smoke. While the problems are common and are found in almost every smoker, there are also a ton of other reasons why you need to quit smoking today.

Alzheimer's Disease

A lot of people do not know this, but Alzheimer's is more common in smokers than in non-smokers because smoking results in mental decline and eventually causes memory loss. Apart from Alzheimer's disease, smokers are also prone to suffer from dementia.

Smoking results in Alzheimer's because of the clogging of the arteries that prevent your brain from functioning effectively.

Autoimmune Disease

Smokers are also at a higher risk of developing lupus which results in chronic pain and inflammation, as well as tissue damage throughout the body. Smokers who quit smoking are less likely to suffer from the autoimmune disease in comparison to those who continue smoking. Patients who have lupus with mild symptoms can increase the severity of the condition by smoking. They can get it treated more effectively when they quit.

Sudden Infant Death Syndrome

Although sudden infant death syndrome is usually related to the position the babies sleep in, about 16% of those deaths were linked to mothers that smoked during their pregnancy. Women who continue smoking when they are pregnant increase the risk of SIDS in their babies. While women believe they had a normal pregnancy and a healthy child, they won't know what can harm their baby.

Tobacco also increases the risk of colic in babies which makes them suffer from severe stomach problems and gastrointestinal issues. These babies are also less likely to reach the desired development milestones at the right age.

Increased Risk of Impotence

While we know that smoking can cause infertility issues in males and females, it is also responsible for erectile dysfunction in men at some stage in their life.

Arthritis

Although most people believe that arthritis is a genetic condition, you can still keep it away even if you have people in your family suffering from arthritis. Arthritis can be kept away as long as you don't smoke. Smoking considerably increases the risk of suffering from rheumatoid arthritis.

Snoring

Smokers tend to snore because of the decreased blood flow to the heart. Even people who are exposed to secondhand smoke end up snoring because it affects them just as much as it affects the person who smokes. One of the major reasons these people smoke is because they are not giving enough oxygen to their lungs because of their clogged arteries due to smoking.

Acid Reflux

Smokers also tend to suffer from acid reflux and heartburn more often as compared to non-smokers. This is because it takes a longer time for the food to digest in the body when there is a high amount of nicotine present and your body does not clean itself as well as you want it to.

Smokers generally suffer from irritability and mood swings as discussed earlier. If you want to lead a healthy life and inhale clean air into your lungs, you should quit smoking and you should make that decision today.

The Effects of Smoking on the Body

Smoking has several side effects on the body because of the high tar and nicotine content. Apart from affecting your lungs, smoking can cause various other problems and the sooner you decide to quit, the less likely you are to suffer from these problems. If you have still not convinced yourself to quit smoking, here are a few symptoms that you need to look out for. These are symptoms that smokers frequently suffer from and may convince you to quit smoking completely.

Mood Swings

Smoking a cigarette is like getting an instant high and while you feel amazing for a while after you have finished smoking a cigarette, you start getting irritable and suffer from anxiety if you stay away from a cigarette too long. This affects your performance and you can't concentrate on getting stuff done without taking a smoke break in between.

Early Menopause

Female smokers are more likely to enter menopause earlier in comparison to non-smokers. Women also tend to suffer from more premenopausal symptoms at a young age because of smoking. Hot flushes are common among young female smokers even when they are far from the age of menopause.

Smelly Hair

One of the worst things about being a smoker is the smell tends to stick to your hair and your body. While you may change your clothes and take a bath every day, if you do not wash your hair, the smell tends to stay there for a long time. Not only is this smell irritating for other people, but it is harmful to your body as well.

Poor Vision

Smoking affects the eyes and also increases the risk of various eye-related diseases, including macular degeneration, glaucoma and cataract.

Bad Teeth

Smokers usually have yellowish and brown stains on their teeth irrespective of how often they go for teeth cleaning session. Smoking weakens the teeth and makes people more prone to infections and inflammation.

Poor Sense of Smell and Taste

The sense of smell and taste is usually dulled out in smokers which is why it decreases the appetite.

Bronchitis

Smokers are more prone to suffer from bronchitis because the smoke constantly affects the respiratory system and this isn't seen in first-hand smokers alone but also passive smokers or secondhand smokers. If you have younger children in the house and a patient suffering from cold multiple times, this could be because of your smoking habits.

Lung Cancer

Smokers are at a significantly higher risk of suffering from lung cancer because of the amount of nicotine that gets accumulated on the lungs. Lung cancer is the most common cancer amongst men and women and the death rate because of this cancer is quite high.

Persistent Coughing

Smokers cough, as it's more commonly called, is something that a smoker suffers from every now and then. This is caused because of the damage to the airways and your windpipe.

Constricted Blood Vessels

Nicotine causes the blood vessels to tighten and this restricts the blood flow. This is one of the main reasons why smokers are at a higher risk of getting a stroke or suffering from frequent high blood pressure.

High Cholesterol Level

Smoking is known to increase bad cholesterol in your body which makes the blood thicker and increases the chances of suffering from a blood clot.

Affects Your Immune System

The immune system of a smoker is generally not as strong as that of a non-smoker which means they are more prone to diseases and they can also contact diseases such as tuberculosis more easily than non-smokers can.

Cervical Cancer

Women that smoke are usually at a higher risk of developing cervical cancer.

Infertility

Men and women who smoke are likely to suffer from infertility issues, some of which could be long term.

Premature Aging

Men and women who smoke tend to get wrinkly skin and even skin that sags a lot faster than those that do not smoke. This is because of the reduced blood flow in your body and your skin not getting enough nutrition.

Cigarettes are easily available everywhere which is why we have a vast population of people smoking them regularly. They contain over 600 ingredients and when burnt they combine to release over 7000 chemicals, most of which are harmful to the body. About 69 of these chemicals are directly linked to cancer which means that your chances of suffering from cancer are a lot higher if you smoke.

The good news is that if you quit smoking, you can reverse most of the side effects within a few years. Begin your journey towards a healthier life and quit smoking today.

Getting Ready to Quit

If you have decided you want to quit smoking it is probably one of the best decisions of your life. In order for you to pull through the plan and ensure that you do not give up midway, it's important to take one step at a time and make sure you follow it precisely. While some people manage to give up smoking fast, there are a few people that require a little motivation and a constant reminder to not go back to smoking. Here are a few ways you should prepare yourself to quit.

Set a Date

If you want to quit smoking, you have to keep yourself prepared to not touch your cigarettes from that day on and the best way to do it is to choose a date and just quit.

Prepare Yourself

If you plan to give up smoking, you need to prepare yourself in advance and this includes getting rid of any cigarettes that you have hidden away and getting rid of your lighters and matchboxes so that you are not tempted to light a cigarette. Things that often remind you of cigarettes are the things that can get your mind diverted towards a cigarette and increase your cravings. To prepare yourself you have to keep those things away. These could be things such as an ashtray or even a metal case for holding your cigarettes. Even if these things hold sentimental value, you need to get rid of them.

Don't Put It Off For Too Long

When you decide you want to quit smoking, choose a date that's really close to the current date. The biggest mistake smokers make is choosing a date as per their convenience and believing that they will be able to give it up if they manage to enjoy these last few days of smoking. Even if a birthday or an anniversary is coming up or even a vacation you want to take, do not let that get in the way of your plans to stop smoking. When choosing a date make sure that the date is no more than a week or 2 weeks away from the day you that you have decided.

Quitting on a Monday

Although we believe that Mondays are blue and stressful, the truth is you are most motivated on a Monday and the chances that you choose to stick to your plan are higher. People who work will find it easier to quit on a Monday because Monday is also the busiest day of the week and you won't even realize you haven't smoked until half the day has passed and this will help keep your motivation level right at the top.

Create a Plan for Yourself

When you decide that you want to quit smoking, make sure you stick to the plan and you are confident about it. Don't second guess yourself and always distract yourself the minute you start thinking of a cigarette. A strong plan can help you to not deviate from your plan and this helps you to go through the week smoothly.

Once you've gone through one week without a cigarette, re-plan every Monday and start afresh so you keep motivating yourself to follow the same routine but you do it with a fresh level of motivation. This works in your favor because you are always excited about it and you also know that you have achieved a certain goal and you're out to achieve even more.

Benefits of Quitting

We have already covered various reasons why you should consider quitting smoking. While we have looked at it from a health issue perspective if you don't quit, let's take a look at the positive things and see how you benefit from quitting and why it is necessary to make the decision soon.

Breaking the Addiction Cycle

When you keep yourself away from cigarettes for a month, most of the nicotine receptors in your brain return to normal and you are on the verge of breaking the cycle of addiction. To put this in simple terms, you overcome the most difficult barrier of quitting and the path to getting nicotine out of your system is relatively easier from now on.

Better Blood Circulation

Once you quit smoking, your body starts to relax and your arteries expand which helps enhance blood circulation. This takes anywhere between 2 to 12 weeks and once your circulation improves the risk of a heart attack decreases considerably.

Better Taste and Smell

Within the first 48 hours of quitting, you realize that you have a better sense of smell and taste and this is something that makes you get back your appetite and enjoy the food you eat.

High Energy Levels

When you quit smoking your energy levels increase because there is an increased level of oxygen in your body and you manage to handle physical activities better.

Boosts Your Immune System

When you quit smoking your immune system gets stronger because of the increased oxygen levels and this helps to lower inflammation. You also manage to fight off colds and other bacterial infections more effectively.

Clean Teeth, Better Breath

When you quit smoking, you are able to look after your dental health a lot better and you will be less prone to oral infections and bad breath. You won't have a sour feeling in your mouth which is common with smokers when they tend to overdo smoking.

Better Sex Life

Smoking can ruin your sex life because it lowers your libido levels. When you quit smoking you will be able to enjoy sex a lot better.

Lower Risk of Cancer

After a few years of quitting you will lower the risk of multiple cancers, including lung, kidney, gallbladder, pancreatic and throat cancer.

How Confident Are You?

When you decide you want to quit smoking, it's important for you to understand how confident you are so you manage to make plans and give up smoking accordingly. Your confidence level doesn't just depend on the number of cigarettes you smoke in a day, but at what times you usually smoke them at and how badly you need a cigarette at that particular hour. Your ability to give up smoking can be decided based on your confidence that you can keep away from a cigarette when you are craving one.

Here is what you need to do. Note down the most common cigarette breaks you take during the day and rate how badly you need to smoke a cigarette at that time on a scale from 1 to 10, 10 should be avoidable and 1 should be very difficult to avoid. Once you have made a list of the timings, you can then plan your day accordingly.

For a lot of people, they need to have their first cigarette in order to go to the bathroom and since this is probably the first cigarette of the day, the craving is probably intense. The rating for smoking this cigarette would be 1 and you need to work hard in order to avoid giving in to this temptation. When you start your day with a positive attitude and you know for a fact that you are going to stop yourself from smoking no matter how bad the urge is, there is a lesser chance you will give up during the rest of the day.

The best way to distract yourself during your no-confidence timings is to do something to keep your mind busy and forget about smoking. If you are used to taking your cigarette with you to the bathroom, try changing your routine and switch to a cup of coffee and read a newspaper during that time. When you have read the newspaper, you automatically divert your mind and you don't think about a cigarette as much as you would if you didn't have anything to do.

Keeping your mind busy doesn't necessarily mean you need to engross yourself in work. Long walks, soothing music or listening to the radio can also divert your mind and help you forget about smoking. If you have a smoking zone inside your house, the first rule should be not to allow smokers or cigarettes inside the house anymore. If you live with roommates and some of them smoke, then you might have to restrict these limits to their bedroom. When you do this, you automatically motivate people around you to make an effort and go outside to smoke. Sometimes they get so busy getting stuff done that they tend to avoid smoking at that time. When you have established no smoking zones around you, there is a lesser chance of giving in to your temptation and your confidence level starts increasing each time.

You should make this list when you start your journey of giving up the addiction completely and revise it every week. You will be surprised to see that your confidence level is continuing to increase as each week passes and before you know it you will have a 10 on 10 confidence for all the times that you craved a cigarette in the past.

Chapter 2 - Planning to Quit

"No-one can quit smoking for you, or make you want to change your life. No-one can make you do anything that you don't want to do." — Gudjon Bergmann

Once you have decided that you want to quit, it's important for you to start planning how you are going to get rid of your addiction in a disciplined manner. You will need a plan because it's not going to be easy. I will say this though, once you get past the first week, it does get a little easier and from then on the journey seems smoother than it was during the first week. Your first week is the make or break period and it's this period that will decide whether you succeed in staying off smoking or you go back to it.

Deciding if You Want to Go Cold Turkey or Using an Aid

Cold turkey is a term that is used for people who give up cigarettes instantly without depending on a nicotine patch or gum to help with their withdrawal symptoms. While some people can use quitting as a medium, others don't benefit from it much and they still have withdrawals even with the aids. When you decide you are quitting smoking, you need to be prepared for common withdrawal symptoms. Some of these include:

- The constant urge to smoke.
- Irritability and anger.
- Headaches.
- Shaking of the hands.
- Constipation.
- Insomnia.
- Dizziness.

While some people suffer from more withdrawal symptoms than others, it's nothing you can't handle once you have decided that you want to quit. The withdrawal symptoms for smokers don't last as long as they do for a drug addict so it's very easy for you to give up the addiction without stressing too much about it and letting it interfere with your routine life.

Identify Your Triggers

While you have a list of the times you like to smoke; you also need to know what triggers the urge to smoke and makes you want to take out a cigarette and light it almost instantly. Different people have different triggers and they also keep changing depending on whether they are weekend triggers or weekday triggers. Your weekly triggers would be the stress at work or the inability to get something done on time, an argument with a loved one or someone in your professional environment or the frequent breaks you take with your colleagues and they all light up a cigarette. Your weekend triggers would either be alcohol and your social life that increases the urge to smoke and peer pressure. While it's easy to deal with your triggers, you have to handle them one at a time and prepare a solution to react effectively for each situation. This will help you to not give in to the urges and face them with confidence.

When you plan on quitting, you have to motivate yourself towards not wanting to smoke anymore. If something triggers the urge, always ask yourself what good will a cigarette do and how is going to help you cope with the situation? Think of an alternative and effective way to deal with the situation and remind yourself that a cigarette doesn't solve anything and it only creates more problems in your life. If you are desperate to smoke and the urge is beyond your control, give yourself time to sit down and relax for a while. Drink a glass of water and eat a small piece of chocolate to help you deal with the situation at hand. Chocolate is a great way to divert your mind and take away the urge of smoking and it also helps to relax your body.

5 Steps of Planning

Quitting can be difficult and it requires a lot of planning in order for it to be successful. Most smokers decide to quit multiple times and end up not being able to do it because something or the other made them light a cigarette all over again and go back to the addiction. If you want to beat smoking like a winner, you have to think like one and stay positive during the process, no matter how difficult it gets. Start slowly but surely and only when you are a 100% sure you are going to give up smoking should you start implementing your plan.

Ignoring External Situations

One of the major reasons why people choose not to quit smoking on a particular date or they decide to quit 2 weeks down the line is because there's something or the other that keeps coming up. You need to remember that birthdays, anniversaries, holidays and parties will keep coming up. If this is going to be the reason for you to postpone your plans to quit smoking, you are never going to do it. When you plan a date and you want to quit smoking, you need to make sure you leave out all the other external factors and focus on the fact that you are going to be able to stop smoking irrespective of what happens from that day on.

Clearing the Clutter

As mentioned before, it is important for you to get rid of anything that reminds you about smoking and apart from your cigarettes and lighters, you also need to make sure you get rid of all ashtrays and the lighter on the dashboard of your car. Another thing you need to do when you decide to quit smoking is to clean your upholstery because that usually starts smelling of stale nicotine and that smell may take you back and increase the urge to smoke again. Make sure you wash your curtains, your bedspread and pillow covers and ensure that nothing remotely smells of cigarettes, so you can quit more effectively. Get your car washed inside out and make sure that the smell of nicotine is gone.

Dealing With Smokers Around You

One of the worst things to deal with when you quit smoking is to face smokers. For the initial few weeks, it is going to be difficult and you will always want to light a cigarette with them. If your friends smoke and they aren't giving up with you, it doesn't mean you have to distance yourself from them. All you need to do is indulge in something that gets your mind off smoking when they are smoking so that you don't crave a cigarette and you can still manage to socialize and be around your friends irrespective of the circumstances. When you are with friends, you could choose to depend on a quitting aid or even choose to simply sip on a juice rather than a cigarette. It will be difficult but once you practice it a few times you'll get used to it and your urge will gradually reduce.

Talk to People

When you quit smoking, it will get a little depressing because it's a tough decision to make and when you do it alone, you often feel left out from your social group of friends because they still continue the habit while you have stopped. Just because you have stopped smoking and the others haven't, it doesn't change anything and the more you talk about your addiction and how you are overcoming it, you will not only manage to motivate others to quit, but you will also let them know how important it is to lead a healthy life. When you talk to people, you don't need to be pushing them or making a decision for them. This is their decision. All you can do is enlighten them with a little information and let them know why it's important to quit smoking and how it could affect their life in the future.

Be Confident

Just because the others haven't quit smoking doesn't mean that they are smarter than you. It simply means it takes them a longer time to understand the importance of healthy living. Quitting smoking is a very smart decision to make and the fact that you have taken the decision shows confidence. No matter what, make sure that you don't fall prey to comments that may instigate you to go back to smoking because that's not going to help you.

Withdrawal Symptoms

Withdrawal is common when it comes to quitting smoking and while quitting immediately may work well for some people, it's not always the solution for everyone because it only increases the urge to smoke in the long run. However, you should know that the best way to quit is to go cold turkey because this is a strong-minded decision and it encourages you to believe that you can give up smoking and stay without a cigarette even if it's for one day at a time. In fact, the best way to look at giving up your addiction is to take it one day at a time, so you don't have to pressurize yourself too much. With regards to the withdrawal, here are a few of the more common withdrawals people face and how you can deal with it.

Nicotine Craving

The sudden urge to go light a cigarette is going to be common for the first few days when you quit smoking and it could be extremely strong in some people while for others it may not be so much. If you were a chain smoker then these withdrawal symptoms may be a little stronger for you because your body will constantly crave the nicotine.

Nicotine craving does not last forever. It comes and goes at the times you usually smoked and they last for about 5 to 10 minutes. While they may not be very strong for some people, for others it could make them extremely uncomfortable and if you are one of those people, then the best thing to do is to sit and relax and start chewing gum or eat a piece of chocolate to subdue the craving. Sometimes long brisk walks also help you overcome this craving.

Snacking and Weight Gain

When you quit smoking, the constant urge to eat more frequently increases, and while a number of smokers who are on the path to getting clean replace cigarettes with unhealthy eating habits and frequent snacks that make them pile on extract kilos, it's always better for you to understand that when you quit smoking, you don't increase your appetite. It just gets back to normal and you should try and satisfy your hunger with healthy meals instead of unhealthy snacking habits. When you eat good food, it reflects well on you and your body starts accepting those nutrients a lot better when you quit smoking and this helps you to get healthy in no time.

Although a smoker tends to put on weight when he or she quits smoking, this only happens because they start eating the wrong food. Healthy eating habits will not make you gain weight so when you plan on quitting, try to keep a lot of healthy food around you to snack in between. This is also a great way to curb the urge to smoke by replacing it with a healthy snack or a fruit.

Sleep Disturbance

The most common side effect of people who give up smoking is sleep disturbance and insomnia because of the lack of nicotine in the body. The good news is you will manage to overcome your sleep disturbances within the first week of quitting but when you do quit and you find it difficult to cope, reduce the caffeine intake and listen to relaxing and soothing music just before you head to bed. Meditation and long walks can help you relax just before you go to sleep and will help you to overcome your sleep problem.

A Persistent Cough

This may seem odd, but when you quit smoking, you start suffering from a persistent cough that is difficult to get rid of. This is because the lining of your airway gets affected when you smoke and when you quit smoking, this lining starts to release all the toxic deposits and starts cleaning your system. This is actually a sign that your body is healing from within. Using cough lozenges and sipping on warm water is a great way to relieve your cough and sore throat. You can add a little honey to warm water to enhance the cleaning process once you quit smoking.

Constipation

Most smokers agree that in order for them to get going in the morning they need a cigarette and when they stop smoking, it is difficult to get the motor running. You need to understand that a cigarette is not a laxative and it does not encourage you to go to the toilet. This is a habit you have set for many years and your body is used to it to release the toxins. If you increase your dietary fiber content, you will realize that you are going more often than you ever did when you were smoking and you don't need a cigarette to get started.

While nicotine withdrawal can be a little difficult to handle, it is nothing that you can't deal with or overcome. When you learn how to overcome these withdrawal symptoms, you will be closer to achieving your goal of saying goodbye to cigarettes for good.

Common Quitting Aids

Although it is highly recommended you quit smoking for long term benefits, some people can't manage to do this and require various quitting aids or smoking aids in order to overcome the addiction. There are different kinds of quitting aids that are available in the market and if you are not confident about going cold turkey then using these aids could help you control the urge to smoke and quit more effectively.

Since there are so many options available, people get confused with regards to what they should choose, but the best way to decide is to give a few of them a try and see which one helps you to curb your craving to smoke more effectively. A common misconception about quitting aids is that it gives you the same pleasure that a cigarette will give you and this is why it disappoints many people. The truth is, while they help you to reduce your withdrawal symptoms to an extent, they in no way pleasure you the way a cigarette would and if you start using them believing that it will replicate smoking then they are not going to work. If you start using them with the belief that they will help curb your withdrawal symptoms, they will prove to be more effective. Here is a list some of the popular quitting aids that you can try.

Nicotine Patches

Nicotine patches are the most common quitting aids people use in order to overcome cigarettes. There are different kinds of nicotine patches available on the market for you to try. Some nicotine patches are strong and can last up to 24 hours and the other ones are a little weaker that work for around 16 hours. If you are a chain smoker then you may want to use the 24-hour patch, so it helps to curb your craving early in the morning, however, if you have a little control on the amount you smoke, then a 16-hour patch can work well.

Nicotine patches release a little nicotine into your system and this can help you to control the withdrawal quite effectively. If you don't want people to know you are trying to quit and you want to control your withdrawal, these patches can be hidden under your clothes. The problem with nicotine patches is that they can cause skin irritation and if you wear them for 24 hours, it could make it uncomfortable for you while sleeping.

Nicotine Inhaler

A nicotine inhaler can work better than a nicotine patch because it releases nicotine vapor straight into your throat which is similar to the feeling of smoking a cigarette. It works relatively faster than a patch and in case you suddenly crave a cigarette, all you need to do is use the inhaler and you will feel fine. The only problem with the nicotine inhaler is it's not very discrete and people around you will notice when you use it.

Nicotine Nasal Spray

The nasal spray is a little stronger than the inhaler and you need to use it by spraying it into each of your nostrils. This spray is highly effective and immediately provides your body with nicotine thereby helping to curb your withdrawal symptoms almost instantly. The nasal spray is one of the only quitting aids that help you to get the rush you experience from smoking. The problem with a nasal spray is it could irritate some people, along with a nose and throat infection and watery eyes.

Nicotine Lozenges

Nicotine lozenges are small tablets that you need to place under your tongue or keep at the side of your teeth in order to curb the withdrawal symptoms you get when you quit smoking. They last longer so they help relax your body more effectively. These lozenges, however, leave a bitter after-taste and don't go down well with everyone. They can last up to 30 minutes and you can keep them in your mouth for as long as you want, but they eventually lose taste.

Nicotine Gum

Nicotine gum has gained a lot of popularity because it not only helps you to curb your withdrawal symptoms, but it also diverts your mind when you start chewing the gum. The gum is available in 2 strengths - 4 mg and 2 mg, depending on how strong your nicotine addiction was. The taste of nicotine gum isn't that great and it leaves you with a fat tongue that often causes difficulty to speak.

Vaping or E-Cigarettes

If you want to replicate the entire process of smoking without the side effects then using e-cigarettes or a vape is something that you can choose to use. While these are highly addictive, they still contain small amounts of nicotine and are not recommended for long term purposes. The problem with e-cigarettes and vapes is that you never get out of the habit of smoking because you are constantly replicating the action of smoking and this makes you more vulnerable to picking up a cigarette and lighting it.

While it is not recommended to use a quitting aid, if you are not confident that you can give up smoking the cold turkey way, you can always choose one of the above mentioned quitting aids and use it on a temporary basis. Try to reduce the dependency on these products and give them up eventually if you want to successfully quit smoking and stay away from cigarettes for the rest of your life.

Dealing with Smoking Triggers

Once you decide you want to quit smoking, you need to make sure you identify the trigger so you can prepare yourself to control the urge of lighting a cigarette. While it seems a little difficult at the start, you will eventually get used to it and you will manage to completely disassociate yourself from smoking and not feel the urge to smoke, even when your triggers are constantly around you. Here are a few triggers that people often relate to when it comes to smoking.

Coffee

Coffee is a major trigger because a lot of people associate coffee and smoking together and because of high caffeine levels in coffee, your body starts to crave nicotine even more. If coffee is a trigger for you, then switch to tea or even a cup of hot chocolate for a while which can help distract your mind from cigarettes and overcome the trigger.

Stress

One of the major reasons why people tend to smoke is because they are stressed and they believe cigarettes can relieve them of their stress. Cigarettes do have a certain chemical that helps people feel relaxed the minute they light it, but these are temporary solutions. The only reason you still want to smoke is because you enjoy doing it. If you are stressed and you can't figure out how to relax yourself without a cigarette, all you need to do is sit back, close your eyes and start taking deep breaths. You can also call your loved one and talk to them for a while in order to distract yourself and make sure that you don't get back to smoking.

After a Meal

Smokers are usually habituated to lighting a cigarette the minute they finish a meal and breaking the habit could get a little difficult when you initially decide you want to quit. The best way to get your mind off a cigarette after a meal is to brush your teeth and have a mint immediately after you finish your meal. When you eat a mint, it helps you to distract your mind from the cigarette and focus on the freshness of the mint. It also makes it easy for you to overcome the urge. If you are at work, try getting back to your work as soon as have you eaten so you can control the urge and if you are at home try washing the dishes to keep your mind off a cigarette.

Boredom

Some people reach out for a cigarette when they are bored and have nothing else to do because it's a habit. If you are one of those people then keeping yourself busy will work wonders. Try downloading a few games on your mobile phone to keep your hands busy so that you don't think about smoking.

Driving

A lot of people tend to crave a cigarette when they are driving and if this is your trigger, then all you need to do is add some beautiful fragrance to your car to get rid of the smoke smell and keep chewing gum and few candies to constantly have something in your mouth while you are driving.

Bars

When you go to socialize with your friends over a drink the chances that people smoke around you are always higher and this could be a strong trigger. Alcohol does lower your motivation level and it makes it easy for you to slip into temptation. If you want to make sure you don't smoke, but you still want to have fun with your friends, try choosing a bar that is smoke-free or if you go to a place that has smokers around, choose to drink something that's not very strong so you can still think rationally. If you are always used to having a glass of whiskey with a cigarette, switch to a glass of red wine so it doesn't remind you of what it tasted like when you had a cigarette.

Sex

Sex is a common trigger for smokers and as soon as they have had sex, they tend to light up a cigarette to continue the high. Instead of smoking after you have sex, try to distract yourself by cuddling with your partner or giving each other massages and talking till you eventually fall asleep.

Bedtime

A lot of people tend to smoke just before they hit the hay and if you are one of those people, then it's very simple for you to overcome this trigger. Simply have a glass of warm milk or try a few meditation sessions to calm yourself down and go off to sleep without thinking about smoking. Reading a book can also help you quit smoking just before you go off to sleep.

Once you learn to deal with regular triggers, it becomes more convenient for you to lead a normal life confidently without thinking about whether or not you are able to cope with the triggers or give in to the temptation.

Checklist - Before You Quit

Once you have decided to go ahead with your plan to quit smoking, you need to get a final checklist to follow and make sure you have ticked off all the pointers before you begin your journey. Make sure that you have everything in place so that you are good to go and you do not let any last minute temptation affect you in any way. Here are a few important pointers:

1. Make sure your home is tobacco-free and free of anything that has anything remotely to do with cigarettes, including lighters and ashtrays.

2. Inform everyone around you so that they don't offer you a cigarette unknowingly and stand in support of your decision.

3. Drink a lot of water and make sure you always have water with you, so you keep yourself hydrated.

4. If you decide on using a quitting aid, make sure you have plenty of it in stock.

5. Keep a lot of gum and mints ready.

6. Get your teeth white and clean.

7. Stock up on a lot of healthy snacks and fruits.

8. Clean up your house and make sure that the smell of tobacco is out of your house for good.

9. Stay away from caffeine beverages such as coffee and soda because this could be very strong triggers.

10. Be confident and believe that you will manage to pull this through.

Chapter 3 - Taking Control

"The best way to stop smoking is to just stop – no ifs, and or butts." - Edith Zettler

Once you decide you want to quit smoking it's important for you to stay focused for the first 2 weeks because this is the critical time period that decides your success or failure. If you manage to stay clean for the first 2 weeks, you will have a higher success rate of giving up smoking for the rest of your life. It's all about taking control and ensuring that the nicotine addiction does not dominate your life and you can make your own decisions without giving in to any kind of temptation. There is a lot at stake during the first 2 weeks because your withdrawal symptoms will be at their peak during these days and your mood won't be at its best. If you want to take control of the situation, you should plan your day in the way that you avoid the triggers completely.

Stay Busy

You often think of a cigarette when you are either doing nothing or when your trigger is activated. The best way to avoid temptation is to keep yourself busy and keep your mind distracted as much as possible. Staying busy doesn't necessarily mean spending long hours at work. You can also plan things with your friends such as a movie or your favorite play or even a sport that you enjoy playing. This is a great time to indulge in a hobby because it helps to keep your mind distracted and it's something that you will enjoy doing. This means you will look forward to doing this every time you think about a cigarette.

You have to remember that no matter how busy you are or how much you distract yourself, the cravings are going to come back to you for the first few weeks and all you can do is sit back and relax and know how to deal with the cravings. Tons of smokers have given up smoking almost a decade ago and still think about what it was like when they smoked but they still don't go back to it. You need to learn to come to an acceptance state where you are proud of the decision you made to quit and it doesn't bother you anymore.

When you initially quit smoking, people who smoke around you will annoy you because it's a constant temptation. After a while, it won't matter whether someone is smoking or not because it's something you choose not to do. You need to train your mind to come to a stage where other people smoking doesn't affect your peace of mind in any manner.

Stay Away From high-risk Situations

During the first 2 weeks, you may want to stay away from high-risk situations where there are a number of smokers because this is the time when you are more prone to giving in to the addiction than ever. You don't have to avoid high-risk situations forever. This will only be for a temporary period till you gain control over your temptations and you are confident enough not to give in just because someone else is smoking. If someone offers you a cigarette, you don't have to be aggressive towards them. You just need to be stern and tell them that you don't smoke anymore and don't intend to do it. Make sure you sound confident when you tell them this, so they don't offer you a cigarette again.

While most of the time people are supportive of your decision, in case you come across somebody who teases you or mocks you for quitting, remind them that it's not something they should be proud of. You need to tell them calmly that you understand the consequences of smoking which is why you decided to quit.

6 Things to do When You Quit

When you quit smoking, you're going to have a lot of ups and downs in life and mood swings play a major role in the process of quitting. When you are constantly reminding yourself about a cigarette, you are in a dark place and this doesn't work well for the process of giving up smoking permanently. If you want to quit smoking with the right attitude, you need to make sure that you mentally prepare yourself and learn to divert your mind every time you think about a cigarette.

Gratitude

This may sound completely irrelevant but the truth is gratitude helps you quit smoking more than anything else. Always learn to be grateful and thankful for the things around you and appreciative of the people in your life. When you learn to be grateful you put yourself in a happy place and when you are happy, you are relaxed. People seldom crave to smoke when they are in a good mood and the more you learn to keep yourself happy, the less likely you are to crave a cigarette. An added benefit to practicing gratitude is that you will start building better relationships with people around you and you never feel lonely. When you quit smoking, there will be scenarios where you feel left out or out of place and when you learn to be grateful, you'll always have people appreciating your presence.

Picture a Healthier You

Every time you think of a cigarette, imagine how your life could be 10 years down the line when you smoke versus 10 years down the line without a cigarette in your hand. Smokers always have certain issues and in most cases, it causes oral irritation each time they smoke. Remind yourself that this could get much worse if you continue smoking. Think about all the side effects that smoking has and how dangerous it is for your body. Keep reminding yourself that you are doing this because your body is your temple and it's your duty and responsibility to look after it for yourself and for your family. Always keep a picture of your loved ones on your office desk so you can remind yourself you are doing it for them.

Keep Your Hands Busy

It is important for you to keep your hands busy because when your hands are busy there is less likelihood of you imagining the entire process of lighting a cigarette and smoking it. You need to remember that while the addiction is because of nicotine running through your body, it is also a little psychological and when you keep your hands busy, there is a lesser chance that you will crave a cigarette in comparison to when your hands are free. If there is nothing to do when you are at home or at work, you can still keep your hands busy simply by pulling out your smartphone and playing a few games to distract yourself.

Read

Reading is a great way to keep yourself busy, not only physically but mentally as well. When you sit in one place with a book in your hand constantly flipping through pages, it is something that engrosses you so deeply that you forget everything else around you. When you choose to read, make sure you pick a subject that interests you and excites you. You may want to stay away from dark fiction, murder and crime because these are the kind of books that will make you feel sad and put you in a dark place. Stick to the kind of books that make you happy, joyful and make your heart sing.

Keep Track of Your Progress

When you quit smoking, you should maintain a journal where you can enter every little detail of your life and what you did to enhance the process of quitting. Write the good, the bad and the ugly in the book because this will help you to express all your thoughts and once you've done, it is out of your system for good. The journal is also a great way to go back and forth and see what triggers these emotions and it will help you figure out how to stay away from them.

Get Moving

The best part about quitting is that you will have a lot of built up energy in your body and you be able to use it in the right way. Try giving your lungs fresh air by going for a walk or even get a small dog, so you have something to look forward to. Since you have decided to quit smoking, you should also try and get a little healthy and indulge in activities that are good for you.

When People Smoke Around You

Just because you quit doesn't necessarily mean everyone around you will quit at the same time and this is something you have to deal with. Remember, you made this decision for yourself and you cannot make it for someone else, but you can surely enlighten them and let them know how bad smoking is. This will help them and the people around them. Make them realize it is always healthy to quit sooner rather than later.

Your Family

When people in the family smoke, especially when there are children around, it increases the risk of infections such as asthma and breathing complications such as shortness of breath, bronchitis and whooping cough. There is a stronger chance children that watch their parents smoke will end up smoking as well because they believe it's the right thing to do since they saw their parents do it. They are also just as prone to ear infections and breathing disorders when people smoke around them and it affects the lungs and heart because of the secondhand smoke. Just because you leave your window open doesn't mean that the smoke is not going to infect others and the sooner you understand this, the sooner you will manage to make a decision.

Your Co-workers

When you quit, you may feel left out or even mocked at times. It's important for you to hold your head high and be proud of the decision you made which is to quit smoking. You can even choose to have an impact on people in various ways. Smoking decreases productivity in a job and it is known to create more complications because of the stress levels and this increases the risk of a heart attack, diabetes as well as other infections. When businesses go smoke-free, they manage to save thousands of dollars because the workers start to be more productive and spend less time on smoke breaks. It also helps keep the environment clean. It is important for one person to take charge and bring in a revolution and if you think you can convince your seniors to create a smoke-free environment at the office, then go ahead and approach them to do it. The farther somebody needs to go to smoke, the less they smoke and this gives them the opportunity to quit as well.

Your Neighbours

Just because they don't live under the same roof doesn't mean that secondhand smoke cannot affect you. When you light a cigarette outside your house, it increases the risk of cardiovascular diseases for all nearby individuals and it also takes a toll on the lungs. The risk of a stroke is also increased by 30% when you are surrounded by people who smoke.

The Good News

- When you quit smoking and make the decision never to go back, it impacts on your own health, heart and lungs and while the secondhand smoke is still bad, your chances of falling ill are still considerably low in comparison to an active smoker. You also help inspire the people around you and when they look at you and see that you've managed to quit successfully, it gives them a ray of hope to try it for themselves.

- If you and your spouse both smoke and you made the decision to quit there is a 67% chance that your spouse will also do the same. You don't have to be married to a person to inspire them. Even a close friend can be influenced by your decision and try to quit.

- The sooner the parents learn to quit, the less likely it is for the children to fall ill and the chances are that they will not smoke in their adulthood.

- When you quit smoking, you have a lot of extra time at work and that time can be put into doing a little more so that you save more money for your family. Let's not forget the expense of cigarettes is now gone and the money can now be saved for something better!

If You Drink Alcohol

Alcohol is not the best thing to have on a regular basis, but if you are a social drinker and you have quit smoking, you can still learn to control your urge to smoke even when you socialize or go out for a drink with friends or family. Just because you have quit smoking doesn't necessarily mean you have to give up on having a social life and since alcohol is one of the major triggers, it is important to learn how to deal with the cravings when you go out for a drink. While you may want to avoid going clubbing or bar hopping with your friends for the first 2 weeks, once you quit it is not something you can put away forever because it's part of you and socializing is healthy. There are a few things you can do in order to control the urge to smoke even when you go out drinking with your friends.

Nicotine Addiction and Psychological Dependence

There are 2 main components of nicotine addiction - one is the physical addiction and the other is the psychological dependence. While the physical addiction is stronger, it's a lot easier to break this addiction and clean your body of the nicotine in comparison to the psychological dependence.

Psychological dependence usually associates smokers with relationships and triggers and this includes the times you need to smoke desperately. If drinking is one of your triggers, then you can always request your friends to visit a bar that is smoke-free so nobody smokes around you and you can control the urge more effectively.

Alcohol Drinking and Control

When you drink too much, you lose your reasoning ability and the ability to control the things that you are tempted towards. This is something you need to keep in mind when you go out drinking. Try to cut down the amount you drink so that you are still sober enough to make the right choices and not give in to the first trigger or temptation that comes your way. You should also try to stay away from the taste of a particular drink that you had along with a cigarette you smoked. This may mean giving up on what you normally drink and switching to something lighter. If you were used to having a glass of beer with your cigarette, try to avoid drinking beer and switch to a cocktail or something a little lighter so you can still focus and have fun but not give in to the urge of smoking.

If You Drink Regularly

If you are a regular drinker, then you may want to cut down on the amount of alcohol you drink because this is not going to help with your goal of quitting smoking. Alcohol has the tendency of breaking your motivation level and getting you in a place where you are most susceptible to give in to an urge. While you don't have to give up alcohol completely, you can still try to control the number of times you drink, so you can give up your addiction to smoking. If you are a social person and you tend to go out very often then the best thing for you to do is switch between alcoholic and non-alcoholic drinks every time you meet people. This will help to curb the addiction and also cut down on the cravings more effectively.

Plan Ahead

If you know you are on the verge of breaking and giving in to an addiction, make an excuse and head to the bathroom or go out to clear your head for a while. When you step outside, make sure not to go too close to people who are smoking because that will increase the urge to smoke. If you know you are going to break, consider calling it a night and head home instead of giving in to the addiction. No matter what you do, do not let alcohol hamper the choice you made to give up smoking and instead of alcohol controlling the situation, you take control of the situation!

If you know for a fact that secondhand smoke triggers you too much, always try to visit smoke-free bars so that you don't witness too many people smoking. While the temptation gets better with time it is always best to make sure you create a strong foundation at the start of your quitting path so that you don't end up giving up easily.

Managing Stress

When you quit smoking, it is a stressful scenario and it is important for you to make sure you learn how to manage your stress levels effectively if you want the plan to be successful. Here are some effective stress-busting strategies that you can apply each time you get stressed out about succumbing to a trigger.

Cut Yourself Some Slack

The fact that you've decided to quit smoking shows that you are aiming to become a healthy person and it is important for you to remember to give yourself credit every now and then. There are going to be little things in and around your life that will keep bugging you and that's the reason you have to clean up the clutter before you make a decision to quit. Along with all the things that remind you about smoking, you should also make sure you have a happy living environment, so you do not fall prey to small distractions and go into a negative mode.

Take Care of Short Term Problems

If you are fighting with friends or family members make sure that you clear the hatchet before you quit smoking because this will trouble you when your withdrawals kick in. Try to talk to as many people as possible because it's important for you to have friends around you when you break the habit of smoking.

Focus on Positive Things

Once you have created a happy atmosphere make sure to focus your energy on things that keep you happy. Try getting plants and focus on looking after your plant or take up gardening. Get yourself a hobby so that you can indulge in doing the things you love and divert your attention to do better and more productive things rather than distracting yourself by getting irritable.

Notice When You Are Stressed

Stress doesn't suddenly come with intense negative emotion, but it creeps in slowly so the minute you realize your slipping into a bad space, start diverting your mind and do something that will keep you happy. Pick up the phone and make a phone call to your loved one or watch a funny video on YouTube just so that you can distract yourself and put yourself back in a good mood.

Do Things You Enjoy

If you are a pet lover, consider bringing home a pet or going to the pet park and watch the animals around. Spend time with nature or maybe consider going out for a trek or going swimming with your buddies. You can also plan a one day picnic with your loved ones where you head out to the park and enjoy a nice meal together.

Managing Highly Emotional Situations

No matter how well you try to keep yourself in a positive frame of mind certain situations may break you and there could also be big triggers to tempt you to start smoking again. Some of these scenarios include:

- A big fight or an argument.

- A financial problem.

- Sudden bad news.

- Losing someone who matters.

- A break-up.

- An emotional setback.

These problems could be a trigger and make you very upset and also push your buttons towards picking a cigarette, but that doesn't mean you should give in to the temptation. You have to keep reminding yourself that no matter how bad situations get, you have to learn to control them and smoking is not the solution. Smoking isn't going to help you feel any better and it's not going to relieve any of the stress you are going through. It only makes matters worse by pushing your body towards being unhealthy. If you want to stay healthy, it's important that you quit and an emotional situation cannot be a trigger for you.

Although you don't see an emotional situation coming up and it suddenly hits you, it's important for you to be mentally prepared for all of the shortcomings because it's part of life and these are all events that will occur in a person's life. If you are finding it difficult to cope with a highly emotional situation, here are a few things that you should try to do.

Let the emotion come out of your system and even if it means crying or waiting for a while for the pain to pass through, let it happen. Do not keep the emotions bottled up inside of you. Try to find somebody to talk to and let it all out of your system because this will help to relieve a lot of stress. You can also write down how you feel in a notebook because this will give you a clear idea of how long it took you to overcome this stress which means if you come across a similar situation in the future, you know how to deal with it. Instead of worrying about what happened, try to look for a solution and plan how you are going to overcome this pain and work towards feeling better.

Staying in Control

After taking control of the situation and you know that you have managed to stay clean for a few days, it's important for you to stay in control so that you don't give in to the urge of smoking ever again. You need to remind yourself that if you could do it for a few days you can do it for the rest of your life and there's nothing that will stop you. It's important for you to learn from your mistakes and make sure you avoid them so that you become smoke-free permanently. Here are some things you should keep in mind in order for you to stay in control.

Don't Be Impatient

The most important thing you need to remind yourself of when you quit smoking is that your body will take its time to get used to the habit of not having nicotine inside the system and this feeling is not going to go away very soon. You have to be patient with yourself and keep reminding yourself how important it is to break the habit and once you manage to break it, you'll never have the cravings again. It's a habit that you've been used to and you have been doing multiple times a day which is why it's not going to go away so easily but once you are done with the first few weeks, it does get easier and this is something that has to motivate you to push yourself every day.

Don't Worry About the Future

When you quit smoking, it's important for you to take one day at a time rather than planning about how well you are going to do a few months later. When you make decisions for yourself months in advance, there is a strong chance those decisions aren't going to work out as planned because you haven't focused on what has to be done today, but rather you try to put in all your energy into planning without realizing whether or not you will be able to curb your urges till then. It's all about making plans on a weekly basis and sticking to them so that you never fail and you manage to achieve all the goals that you wanted to achieve during the week. This will also help with your motivation levels. You can put up a chart in your home or your office that will track your progress and see how you managed as a non-smoker. You can even make note of the money that you saved when you did not purchase cigarettes. This will keep you going.

Don't Be Negative

When you quit smoking, there are going to be feelings of negativity that will keep coming up and you start feeling low and depressed. You have to stay strong every time a temptation comes and you have to try to tell yourself that you have what it takes to quit and this is the feeling you never need to let go of. Keep giving constant reminders to yourself that you are stronger than this and you will manage to quit. Start reading positive quotes and keep telling yourself that you are strong enough to do this and you will go through the journey successfully.

Don't Neglect Yourself

It is important for you to focus on your health when you quit smoking because there are a number of factors that may enhance your hunger and make you want to eat unhealthy food.

Eat Healthy

Instead of eating unhealthy snacks, make sure to keep healthy snacks ready for you all the time because not only does this help to keep you full, it will help to get rid of all the dirty toxins of cigarettes that are stored in your system. Always keep healthy fruits and nuts ready so that you can munch on them when you are hungry. Make sure to eat frequent small meals rather than large ones because this helps to keep your body's metabolism high and prevents weight gain when you quit smoking.

Rest Well

When you quit smoking, you may have trouble sleeping and the best way to learn how to overcome this issue is to meditate just before you head to bed or drink one glass of milk. Not only will this help you relax your nerves but it also helps to subdue a trigger in case you have a habit of smoking just before you head off to sleep.

Drink Water

It's important for you to hydrate your body when you quit smoking because it's a great quitting aid and it not only helps to control the temptation of smoking, but it helps cleanse your system from within, thereby getting rid of all the dirty nicotine and tar accumulation inside your system. If you can, try having a warm glass of water with honey each morning because honey is rich in antioxidants and it is also a great healing agent.

Take a Multivitamin

Cigarettes drain your body of all the necessary nutrients and this means that your body is probably lacking a lot of the vital nutrients required for its management. Consult your doctor and ask your doctor to provide you with a good multivitamin that can help you gain a lot of energy and keep you strong during the process.

Limit Alcohol Consumption

While an ideal scenario would be to quit alcohol completely, if you can't do this, you can still try to limit the amount of alcohol you drink so that you can stay healthy and cut down the temptation of smoking. Alcohol is one of the major triggers and it is no secret that people tend to smoke more when they drink, so you have to figure out the best possible way for you to keep your temptation in control in case you plan on having a drink.

Don't Overdo It

While it is important that you stay focused for the first few days, it doesn't mean you get so strict with yourself you forget having fun. You have to learn a balanced way to enjoy the process of quitting rather than making it a stressful one because this is a plan that will not work if you are stressed. You should set weekly goals and for every goal, you achieve you should reward yourself with something small. Try to keep the end plan as a big gift for yourself and give yourself a year to do it. If you have purchased a pack of cigarettes every day make sure to put that amount of money aside for your end goal, so you are more motivated towards it. This will help you to enjoy the process and will also give you something to look forward to.

Don't Hesitate to Ask For Help

If you believe that you need to talk to somebody or you need advice, make sure that you go and get that help as soon as possible. A lot of times people just don't know what to do and how to take the next step which is why they give up midway when they could have easily spoken to somebody about the problem. Whether you talk to a loved one or you try to get in touch with people who have quit smoking, it's always good to reach out because this helps you go through the journey a lot more conveniently. When you ask people for help, it eases the pressure as they also know what you are going through and they will tell you whether or not it's normal, so this gives you more motivation.

Don't Think You Can Smoke Just One Cigarette

When you quit smoking, there's no such thing as smoking just one cigarette as an excuse because that is a sign you are never going to quit. You either go cold turkey, or you use a quitting aid, but you should not go back to cigarettes and this is a decision you have to make if you want to stay in control. Once you give yourself a leverage to smoke one cigarette, you will want to keep going back and this is not going to help you.

Remind Yourself Why You Quit

Everyone quits for a reason and you need to keep reminding yourself why you did it and why you need to stay away from the temptation every day. Your reason to quit is your main motivation and it is something that will make you stay away from smoking so keep reminding yourself why you did it and why you need to stick to your plan.

Chapter 4 - What About Weight Gain?

"It is in your moments of decision that your destiny is shaped." –Tony Robbins

One of the major reasons why people choose not to give up smoking is because they are afraid of gaining weight. This is something that's obvious and as much as one would like to ignore it, it is a known fact that a person who quits smoking has the tendency of gaining more weight because of a number of factors.

The Reason People Gain Weight After Quitting

Let's be honest; smoking does increase metabolism rates a little which means that a smoker can burn up to 200 calories if they are going through about a packet of cigarettes a day. Nicotine also works as an appetite suppressant which means you tend to eat smaller meals when you smoke.

When you quit smoking, most people tend to gain around 10 pounds in the first few months which is normal. However, if you don't control your eating habits, you may gain more weight which is why it's important for you to understand the effects of quitting and handle them with caution.

Why Do You Eat More

Smoking is an appetite suppressant and this simply means that when you quit, you start feeling more hungry and end up eating larger meals. Smokers usually pull out a cigarette and smoke every time they get a break instead of eating a snack and this kind of keeps them pumped up. When you stop smoking your body craves for something and the next replacement that non-smokers find is food, which is why they start to feel more hungry.

While it's not wrong to replace food with a smoking habit, it's important for you to understand what kind of food you are replacing it with. Most non-smokers tend to just binge on unhealthy snacks such as wafers and chips that come packed with calories and directly contribute to weight gain. They also switch to tetra pack sweet fruit juices that have a lot of sugar and are not going to do you any good. While a good appetite is a good thing, it is important for you to feed your body healthy food for the appetite to benefit your body rather than destroy it.

Understand the Difference Between a Good and Bad Snack

If you want to stay healthy when you quit smoking you have to figure out what is healthy for your body and what is not so that you keep control of what you eat. Instead of feeding your body with junk, substitute it with healthy alternatives that benefit your body and also help to cleanse it rather than gain weight. Smokers are usually underweight, so when you put on a little weight it's fine, but once you've reached your normal weight, you should try and eat food that is healthy for your body so that you maintain the weight.

You should also be on the lookout for snacks that help boost your metabolism because it's important for you to feed your system something that can keep your digestive system up and running. Another important thing you should do is to frequently have a snack that is healthy instead of eating unhealthy meals 2 to 3 times a day. Even your big meals should be small in proportion and should be focused on healthier items such as vegetables and lean meats rather than unnecessary carbohydrates and calories. You should also try to stay away from aerated drinks that are loaded with sugar that people usually use to accompany their meal with. The reason a person who has just quit smoking has a liking towards these aerated drinks is because they have caffeine which is one of the ingredients present in a cigarette. When you understand what you should eat and how you can keep your system healthy, you will manage to balance your weight and not gain too much during the process of quitting.

Exercise

If you want to stay healthy and you want to make sure your metabolism rate is still effectively high, it is important you exercise on a regular basis. Exercising is good for your body and it also keeps you active and helps your organs function better. A simple brisk walk for 30 minutes is perfect on a daily basis and you don't have to really go to a gym or struggle with intense workouts to stay in shape.

Avoid Too Much Alcohol

Alcohol has a lot of calories and it can immediately make you put on weight in all the wrong places which is why you may want to cut down on your alcohol intake if you want to get fit. When smokers drink alcohol, they burn calories because of the amount they smoke during the drinking session and once this stops these calories are going to get accumulated in your body. Alcohol also happens to be a very intense trigger for smoking so try keeping it to a minimum as far as possible.

Deal With One Challenge at a Time

There is no denying that weight gain can often bring about frustration and demotivate you during the process of quitting but that doesn't mean you give in to those feelings and let go of your plan to give up smoking. You need to deal with one problem at a time for the first 2 weeks and you have to put your complete focus on quitting the habit of smoking so that you are able to then focus on keeping yourself healthy. You have to learn to be patient because it's important for you to understand what's going on in your body for you to take control and stay in control. Don't let negative thoughts affect you and don't let what people say make a difference in your life because you are in control and you shouldn't let anybody else tell you what's good and what is not.

While it is important to be kind to yourself, you need to understand no matter what, you should love yourself. If you are gaining a little weight to give up a bad habit is something that you have to put up with, you need to handle it in a way that you will manage to deal with positively rather than feel bad about it.

Understanding Relapses and Slips

Relapses and slips are common when you quit smoking, but it doesn't mean that you give up and forget why you chose to quit in the first place. It's important for you to identify whether it is a relapse or a slip and how you need to deal with the situation. Here is what you need to know about relapses and slips.

Relapse

A relapse is referred to as something that happens to you when you decide you are going to stay off cigarettes for a few days and then go back to smoking your regular way. The stages are usually something like this:

- You give in to a temptation and purchase a pack or smoke a cigarette from a friend.

- Feel guilty about smoking and start blaming yourself.

- Tell yourself that you can't quit and you go back to smoking.

- Give up on the plans of becoming a non-smoker.

A Slip

A slip is referred to as something that happens to you when you smoke a cigarette or take a puff and immediately go back on track by staying clean. The stages look something like this:

- You take a puff, or you smoke a cigarette.

- You give up midway smoking an entire cigarette and then tell yourself that it's wrong and you have to give up this habit.

- Find a new way to deal with temptation.

- Never touch a cigarette again.

- Keep going.

You have to remember that every slip does not necessarily mean it goes into a relapse and it's from these small mistakes you make that you will eventually succeed. All you have to do is keep trying.

Stop the Slide

It is common to have a slip or 2 during the process of quitting, but you have to figure out how not to make a habit out of it because then this is a relapse that is hanging on thin ice and ready to kick in the minute you have a big trigger or an emotional setback. Whether you are going cold turkey or using a quitting aid, you need to keep reminding yourself smoking is wrong and even if you take a puff, it's a big mistake that you have made and why not to do it again. However, you need to learn when to forgive yourself and move on rather than just keep pondering on the thought and feeling bad about it because this will just make you feel like you can never quit and you'll eventually go back to smoking permanently.

There will be times when you believe that you are just too stressed out and it's not working but those are the turning points in your life and if you pull through those milestones you will manage to get stronger.

You Have to Learn to Trust the Process - The Process of Quitting

Quitting a cigarette is similar to that of a child learning to ride the bicycle. You are going to fall down or put your foot down to get the balance right, but that doesn't mean you give up. If you put a cigarette to your lips it's like you put your foot down and if you take a puff, it is like you falling off the cycle, but that doesn't mean you don't get on and try again. Remember the more often you try, the less likely you are to fall and break the habit again or relapse and it's all about just keeping faith and going on even when it's difficult for you to cope.

The True Problem

You need to realize why you slipped in the first place and what made you give in to a cigarette after all the efforts that you have put into staying clean. Sometimes triggers are underlying and you need to identify them instantly which is why you need to take the time to see what caused you to slip so that you ensure it doesn't happen again.

A non-smoker for Life

When you decide to quit smoking, you have to make a choice of whether you want to be referred to as an ex-smoker or a non-smoker. While people believe there is no difference between them, since you've always been smoking, you would be referred to as an ex-smoker and not a non-smoker. The truth, however, is what you refer to yourself as plays a huge impact on how you are going to plan your future. A non-smoker is someone who is never going to smoke and not someone who has never smoked in their life and an ex-smoker is someone who has smoked in the past and may go back to smoking every now and then when they come across an emotional setback or a trigger. You have to make a decision to stay a non-smoker for the rest of your life if you want to get the benefits of quitting smoking. While it is healthy for you to give up smoking, there are also some added advantages that people often forget about.

You Feel Great

For the first few weeks, you will feel terrible and that's not a fact I want to hide because if you go in with the mindset that the process is easy, you will give up the minute it gets difficult. If you go in with the mindset that this is not an easy path to take, but you still are going to take it, there are less chances you will break! However, once you get over the first few weeks life feels a lot better and you start getting healthier. You sleep a lot better, you tend to eat better and you taste food more effectively. Your sense of smell comes back and the best thing about quitting is that you get rid of the irritating and pestering cough in your throat.

You Lead a Cleaner Life

When you smoke the smell of cigarettes starts lingering around your atmosphere such as your home, in your car or even in your office smoking zone and that's not a pleasant smell to deal with. While you were so used to the smell you didn't know how bad it was, you should ask a non-smoker and they will tell you just how disgusting that smell can make them feel. That lingering smell can affect you in more ways than you could imagine and apart from shortness of breath and irritation, it is also responsible for a chronic cough that happens from time to time. When you give up smoking, you get rid of all the dirty smells and you live in an environment that's more positive and smells better. Let's not forget smokers have smokers' breath and they also smell really bad. When you give up smoking, you feel more confident, especially when stepping into an air-conditioned room because there is no longer a smell that you carry with you.

You Save Money

It is an obvious fact that people who smoke spend up to $10 a day on cigarettes, that amounts to a staggering $3000 in a year! Imagine the things you can purchase with that money. Start saving today and one year down the line when you have enough, you can make use of it in a more effective way by getting yourself something that you can call a reward for staying off cigarettes for so long.

Chapter 5 - Friends and Family

"At least three times every day take a moment and ask yourself what is really important. Have the wisdom and the courage to build your life around your answer." - Lee Jampolsky

When you plan on quitting it is important that you inform your entire family and keep them in the loop because their support matters and when they know what you have decided to do, they will support you 100%. People that actually matter to you will be glad to hear that you have decided to quit smoking and they will make sure they make the environment as comfortable as possible for you which is why sharing is important.

When you realize that you have an addiction to smoking and you have decided that you are going to change, then it will definitely be something that works in your favor. When you start getting tempted to light a cigarette, there's always somebody there to stop you and assure you that you can do it.

When you have family and friends that support you, there are various things that you can do to enhance the quitting process. When family and friends are involved your break time becomes easier to deal with because people know that you are not smoking and they try to not smoke in front of you to encourage you with your decision. This is considered to lower the risk of triggers in your life and it makes you feel confident. While approval from others is not necessary, the motivation that comes from them surely helps you to feel better and makes the journey a lot easier. The important thing to remember when you give up smoking is to not force others to do the same just because you've made the decision. If they are supporting you with your choices, you need to be fine with the choices they make as well. Just because your friends haven't given up smoking yet doesn't mean you start lecturing them about the side effects of smoking, on how bad it is and set yourself as a superior example in front of them because this isn't going to help them in any way. They are supportive of you and if you silently go on with the process, they might be inspired and make the decision for themselves sooner or later. However, this is not something you can make for them or tell them to do. You need to reflect back at the time you made the decision and you will realize that at the end of the day, you realizing was all that mattered and no matter what all the people said, you still continued your habit till you decided to give up on your own.

While it is good to tell people how you did it, you don't have to tell them when to do it. If you really want somebody to quit smoking, you have to give them the space and time to prepare and set a living example rather than be a preacher.

4 Steps to Helping

When you decide you want to quit smoking you have to make your choices the right way so that it works well in your favor. There are various decisions you have to make, but there are 4 essential steps that will help you stay on track and ensure that you do not lose focus of what you are doing and why you are doing it in the first place.

Write Down Why You Want to Quit on a Card or Save it on Your Mobile Phone

This card is referred to as your motivation card and the reason you quit has to be something strong because this is the reason that will stop you from smoking every time you want to go back. If you have kids they should be your focus because there's nothing a parent won't do for their child and giving up smoking is just a speck of dust in comparison to the leaps and bounds that a parent is willing to go to for the child. Even if you are single, look at yourself in the mirror and tell yourself that you are beautiful and your life is worth living and you are not going to abuse your body by smoking and destroying your body one day at a time. The reason it's important for you to have this written down is that every time you look at it, you will remind yourself of how important the decision you made is and it will stop yourself from slipping or relapsing.

Tell Yourself it is Going to be Easy

It might not be the easiest thing to do, but you have already made the toughest decision which is to quit and nothing can be more difficult than deciding you're going to give up smoking. So from the day you smoke your very last cigarette, you have already won half the battle because you had the motivation and the courage to curb the urge which means you have what it takes to go to the end. Instead of keeping long gaps and planning your day well in advance, do it on a weekly basis so you can keep rewarding yourself when you do something good and when you have achieved your goal. As a smoker, it is difficult to do a lot of physical activities and this includes working or going up a flight of stairs. Keep thinking of the things you couldn't do when you smoked and attempt them so that you motivate yourself better and you see the progress inside of you. Positivity is important when you quit and reading motivational quotes and messages every now and then will definitely help keep you going and stop you from smoking.

Note Down Your Progress

It's important for you to maintain a journal and keep track of everything you do right from the day you started your journey towards a smoke-free life. Write down what was the temptation, how you feel and the little accomplishments you have achieved along the way so that you keep yourself going and you are always motivated. Make sure to keep this journal with you no matter where you go so when you are feeling low you can just flip through the pages and look at how much you have already managed to do. This can help you stop the deepest temptation and say no to cigarettes when you want them the most.

Detoxify Your System

If you have been a smoker for a long time there a lot of toxins that are built up in your system and it's important for you to start the cleansing process when you quit smoking. There are simple things that you can do, including consuming a lot of natural products to help heal and clean your body. Herbal teas, vitamins, amino acids and antioxidants are some of these things that you can get at your local medical store, or you could choose to have them fresh through fruits and vegetables.

Why It's Hard to Quit Smoking

Honestly, it's not easy to give up smoking and most people who try, fail for the first time and never try giving up again. There are a few who keep trying it on a regular basis but with a lot of ups and downs during the course. A lot of smokers feel proud in saying they can't give up because they are addicted and it's too difficult.

To begin with, smoking is not something you should be proud of. It is harmful for your body, it affects your mind and it pollutes the environment. The minute you start telling yourself these things you will want to quit no matter how proud a smoker you are! When you see a group of people smoking, it's not cool. They are making a mistake and for many years advertising and media have been responsible for this. If you quit smoking, you are not going to become a cool person, or you're not going to be labeled as a boring person who doesn't like to have fun. These days, a lot of youngsters are quitting cigarettes because they believe that their health is more important. Apart from cigarettes, there are a lot of other addictions have been introduced including harmful drugs and people these days believe that it's great to keep trying them because all their friends are doing it and it makes them feel good. But when you try it once, it turns out to be an addiction that you struggle with for a really long time until you finally make a decision to quit. Unlike other drugs, giving up smoking can get difficult and here is why.

According to a recent survey, only about 7% of people who attempt to quit smoking can successfully do it in the first try and do it when they go cold turkey. That doesn't mean you can't be part of that 7%. All you need is a strong plan and motivation in order for you to go through the entire process without turning back. Yes, your body will crave nicotine and you will suffer withdrawal symptoms but this is nothing that you can't deal with and in case your irritation and depression is a little high, always depend on playing games. When you give up smoking for good, your withdrawal symptoms start to fail and once you are done with the first 2 weeks, they almost disappear and the only thing that remains is the temptation that you may want to go back to smoking. If you have that under control, you won't go back.

It's Not Just About Willpower

You may think you have willpower, but apart from willpower you also need to be in a happy place and stay positive all the time. No plan is designed to succeed the first time and if you do have a slip, it doesn't mean that you are going to be a smoker for the rest of your life. It just means you need to try a little harder and focus on what triggered you to fall into the temptation so you can avoid it.

Some people achieve success when they try the first time while others need to try it multiple times and with a little extra effort and determination you will become a non-smoker in no time.

How People Quit Smoking

If you want to quit smoking the one thing you need to understand is that this is a lengthy process and there are no shortcuts. Just because you stayed clean for 3 days doesn't mean that you have overcome your addiction. It takes a long time for your mind and body to get over the effects of smoking and even after 2 or 3 months you may still feel a strong urge to smoke, especially if there is a negative or emotional setback. This is why you need to do it the right way in order to lower the chances of failure.

While you may have understood how important it is for you to identify your triggers and deal with them, you also need to make sure that you learn to cope with your triggers over a period of time so that they don't affect you for the rest of your life. Instead of trying to run away from your triggers you need to make yourself strong enough to face them and understand that no matter what the circumstances, you will never go back to smoking.

You need to have a strong will power to give up smoking, but that's not the only thing. When people go cold turkey, only 7% of them succeed and if you were a chain smoker, it is going to be really difficult for you to cut out cigarettes completely without you slipping or relapsing. It's important for you to understand how comfortable you are with the situation and accept if you need help with quitting aids that can help you overcome the triggers. Once you start using a quitting aid, you can always learn to cut down the number of times you use it till your body recovers completely. It makes more sense to use something that helps you cope with the addiction rather than getting frustrated and wanting to give in to every trigger that crosses your path.

You need to understand what withdrawals are like and figure out what your withdrawal symptoms are in the first place. We already know the signs of withdrawals but that doesn't mean that everyone suffers from the same ones. It is different for different people and while some may just have a headache, others may have difficulty sleeping. Once you identify your withdrawal symptoms, it becomes easy for you to treat them and use them rather than getting irritated and annoyed each time you feel that way.

Irritation is common and it happens to almost everybody who gives up smoking. The thing about meditation is this is going to last you forever and after the first 2 weeks you tend to forget these signs altogether and you become a generally happy person. Smokers suffer from mood swings and once you cross the 2 week mark, these mood swings and other signs of depression slowly disappear.

You need to understand the various facts about smoking as well as about quitting so that you have a clear mind and you don't simply trust what people say. Giving up smoking may be tough, but it's not impossible and with the right guidance you will manage to do it successfully.

Chapter 6 - Other Tobacco Products

"It's gonna get harder before it gets easier. But it will get better; you just gotta make it through the hard stuff first." - Unknown

Cigarettes are most common when it comes to tobacco products, but there are also other tobacco products available on the market that are harmful to the body and need to be avoided. When we normally say that the risk of tobacco is associated with smoking, people that are addicted to other tobacco products usually tend to ignore these facts. Here is a list of the other tobacco products that are harmful and also need to be stopped if you want to lead a healthy life.

Cigars

Cigars are normally considered to be a statement of style and class and it's something only the rich people use on a regular basis. Cigars are not very different from cigarettes because they also have tobacco inside them. The only difference between a cigarette and a cigar is that a cigar is larger than a cigarette in terms of size and it's wrapped in tobacco leaves rather than a paper.

A cigar tastes very different when compared to a cigarette and for those who are not used to smoking a cigar will find it very annoying and irritating because it hits the throat directly. Cigar smoking is just as harmful as cigarette smoking and if you thought that it's a safer way to keep your nicotine addiction up, you couldn't be more wrong. People who smoke cigars are still likely to suffer from various cancers including the lung, the oral cavity and the larynx. Cigar smoking is one of the leading causes of erectile dysfunction in men.

Pipes

Pipes and cigars are similar to each other when it comes to side effects and these are just as harmful. Pipes use raw tobacco that's inserted inside the pipe to smoke. These were really popular back in the day and were available in large numbers before cigarettes became popular. Pipes seem to have become more popular these days not only because of tobacco smoking but also with various other drugs that people smoke. When you use a pipe to smoke, you take in the smoke directly to your lungs which increases the risk of lung cancer. Cigarettes have filters while pipes don't and this means that all the nicotine and tar enters your system directly when you smoke through a pipe.

Smokeless Tobacco

Smokeless tobacco is available in packets and people need to sniff it or rub the tobacco between the cheeks and the gums. This is probably the worst form of tobacco because it is high-risk and it causes various problems including an extremely high-risk of mouth cancer. This form of tobacco is banned in a number of places because of the side effects. It's the most difficult of all the addictions to give up because it gives you an instant high. Smokeless tobacco must be treated seriously and if you use it on a regular basis, you need to take into consideration the serious consequences and quit it today.

Quitting Smoking While in Recovery

Not a lot of people know this, but there are rehabilitation centers that can help you get over your addiction with cigarettes as well as tobacco. While it's not necessary for you to enroll in the center, you can always give it a try to help with your addiction more effectively. The stay in these centers is relatively short and once you are done with your first 2 weeks, they usually let you go. These are not the kind of centers where you have to stay inside, but it is a self-check-in where you go to get treated at your own will. The word rehabilitation may seem to be a bit negative and a lot of people refrain from entering the centers because they believe they will be labeled as an addict or something worse. If you were trying not to go into a rehabilitation center even though you know your smoking addiction was really bad, it's important for you to understand that a rehabilitation center doesn't necessarily mean you have a problem. It simply means you are strong enough to address your problem and this is what you have to tell everyone around you.

There are benefits of getting yourself enrolled in a center to quit smoking because when you do this, you leave no room for error and it simply means that you will have to give up irrespective of what withdrawals you go through or how you feel. This is an extreme step to take but if you are not confident enough and you know you won't be able to give it up on your own, taking the step may not make a lot of sense. Smoking is more dangerous than alcohol and if people can get enrolled in a center to get over alcohol addiction, there is no shame in getting into a center to overcome smoking. The side effects of smoking are more severe than alcohol is, so do it and do it right to treat yourself and get healthy.

Another reason why people try to stay away from a rehabilitation center is that they believe that once they are outside, they may get into the addiction all over again. If you are going cold turkey and you are being assisted by a rehabilitation center your chances of success are much higher than when you do it independently. The reason being when you are in a rehabilitation center, their professionals are present in the center to ensure you are not attracted to cigarettes or you don't have the slightest reminder of it. They do this for the first 2 weeks which are the most difficult days to deal with post quitting.

In the rehabilitation center, they teach you the various ways to overcome your triggers and not give in to temptation and make you strong enough to deal with anything that is thrown in your face to ensure you never touch a cigarette again. People who enroll for rehabilitation centers are also less likely to relapse or slip even once after they have given up smoking because they get so strong and they feel confident about their decision. While it's not compulsory for you to enroll in a rehabilitation center in order for you to overcome your addiction, it is something you can definitely consider if you are not confident doing it on your own.

Chapter 7 - Why People Use Tobacco

"Our strength grows out of our weakness." - Ralph Waldo Emerson

Cigarettes gained a lot of popularity back in the 1920s and ever since, the demand for cigarettes and the number of smokers has kept on increasing. It is difficult to understand why something so bad for you gained so much popularity and how it is still legal. Here are some facts about cigarettes and why it is so difficult to get over the addiction.

It Makes You Feel Free

Cigarettes were introduced onto the market with a very positive influence and some leading actors and actresses supported a campaign that promoted smoking. Not just men but women also felt liberated by smoking and proved that it's something everyone should do to feel free and good. Once this became a trend, it became difficult for people to give up and more and more people started getting addicted to smoking. Back in the day, people weren't even aware of the side effects of cigarettes so much so that doctors recommended it.

Social Acceptance

One of the leading reasons why people still smoke is because they want to feel socially accepted by a crowd. It is difficult to find a group of teenagers that don't smoke today and when you try to stay away from smoking, you either feel left out or are treated differently. With an aim to get close to friends, people make sure that they smoke around everyone so that they are a part of the group.

Sophistication

Smoking is considered as an act of class, elegance and sophistication and most movies and advertisements represent the highest statute of society smoking which is what influenced a large number of people to get into the habit. So much so that cigarette companies started designing slimmer looking cigarettes to look elegant in the hands of a woman. By 1960 the popularity of a cigarette grew so much that almost every second person was smoking.

Celebrity Influence

Celebrities have posed with cigarettes for a really long time and you still often spot pictures of celebrities with cigarettes in their hand. People who look up to the celebrities as role models often believe this is what they should do in order to look and feel like them.

Weight Loss

One of the major reasons people, especially women, continue to smoke is because it helps to maintain a slim structure and they know for a fact they won't gain weight when they continue smoking. It's a small price they believe they are paying to stay fit, but the truth is when you follow a healthy lifestyle you will still manage to stay fit even when you quit smoking.

Peer Pressure

The main reason people start smoking is because of the pressure of society and once they start smoking, it gets really difficult for them to give up the habit. What you believe is cool during your school and college days eventually turns out to be something that does not benefit you for the rest of your life. Giving up smoking is a difficult task to do and it is easier to say no before you even start.

It is also important for you to make your children aware of the bad side effects of smoking and how harmful it is to the body. You need to teach them that it's not necessary for them to give in to peer pressure and do what they know is wrong just to fit into the crowd. If your child understands the importance of staying healthy and staying away from cigarettes, they won't fall prey to what society has to say. It's also important for parents to set an example for their children by not smoking themselves. If you tell your child that smoking is bad, but you smoke in front of your child, it's not going to be a very good example for them.

Coping Mechanism

People believe that cigarettes help to relieve a lot of stress and that is far from the truth. You need to stay strong if you want to give up an addiction or not give in to it at all. Hiding behind the cloak of a cigarette to get relief from stress is not going to get you anywhere. People who feel low or hurt for some reason often turn to a cigarette to get some sort of comfort. The truth, however, is cigarettes will only give you temporary relief and it is not going to heal you in any way. The only way you will be able to get out of a negative state of mind is when you seek help and let people know how you truly feel.

Cigarettes are never the answer to anything and it can never benefit anyone in any way and the sooner you realize this, the more effectively you will be able to live your life.

Whether you have been smoking for a few months or whether you have been a smoker for most of your life, it doesn't matter! What matters is taking the right decision today and deciding that you want to quit and never turn back and light another cigarette in your life.

Common Myths

When it comes to quitting there are a number of questions that run through your mind. There is also some things people will tell you to discourage you from quitting and make you believe that you should continue smoking. Here at 10 smoking myths that we have busted for you so you can make your decision with a clear head.

It Causes Weight Gain

While quitting can help you increase your appetite and enable you to eat more food, it doesn't necessarily mean it will cause weight gain. If you want to stay healthy while quitting all you need to do is focus on eating the right kind of food and you won't put on any weight. Although smokers are generally below weight, giving up the addiction doesn't mean you will gain a lot of weight instantly. It simply means you will get healthy as long as you focus on eating the right food instead of unhealthy junk food. Just like smoking, unhealthy food is also an addiction that you need to refrain from once you quit smoking. A little exercise and the right diet will not only help you to keep your weight in control, but it will also make you a healthier person.

It Promotes Mood Swings

You will get a little agitated when you quit smoking but this is something that doesn't last for a long time and within the first 2 weeks you overcome your mood swings naturally. Even when the mood swings happen, they are not permanent and it generally goes away within the first 10 to 15 minutes of it being triggered. The reason you're getting these mood swings is that your body is adjusting to not having nicotine in the system and it's a good sign because it shows you are on the road to recovery. If you find that the mood swings are severe, you can always switch to using nicotine aids in order to keep them in control and still manage to get over the withdrawals gradually. You need to remember that when you quit smoking, it's not something you do immediately but something that takes a while for your body to adjust to and the more comfortable you make yourself during the process, the higher the chance of success is.

You Will Get Depressed

People believe that mood swings and depression are a part of the quitting program but it's actually not. Depression is usually an underlying issue that you try covering up when you smoke but this isn't a permanent solution and when you give up smoking it might seem a little more prominent to you. If you know you are depressed, it makes more sense for you to get yourself treated rather than letting it bother you and letting it get in your way. You need to remember that when you give up smoking, it doesn't cause depression. It just makes you a little irritable because of the nicotine craving in your body. Depression and sad feelings are something that come from within and you need to address it in a different way to figure out why you are having these feelings in the first place.

It Will Ruin Your Social Life

If you are a strong person and you make the right decisions for yourself quitting is not going to affect your social life in any way. While you may need to refrain from your triggers for a while once you quit, you don't have to do it permanently. You can always go back to your routine social life once you know you won't get tempted to smoke. You can also plan fun activities with your friends and your loved ones that don't involve smoking in any way or going close to places that trigger your instinct to smoke.

You Lose Your Friends

If you are a smoker, the chance that your friends are also smokers is high and this is often a fear that people have when they give up smoking. Honestly, if your friends really care about you, they may also consider giving up smoking with you rather than force you to get back to the habit. No matter how old you are or how young you are, taking a decision to quit is something that will have a positive impact on everyone and they will eventually realize how good it is to stay smoke-free. When you make your decision just make it with confidence and announce it to your friends by humbly requesting for their support. A good friend will always stand by you in your decision and will never you go the wrong way.

You Won't Be Creative

Addiction to smoking and creativity goes a long way and creative people often fear that if they stop smoking, they won't be able to unleash their creativity the way they used to. Let's look at this from another perspective.

Smoking negatively affects your brain and it disturbs the ability to think! If you were creative when you used to smoke, imagine how creative you'll be once you quit. Creativity has nothing to do with smoking and if anything, giving it up will help enhance your creative skills because you will be more focused and you have more energy in you.

You Will Develop A Cough

You may get a cough when you quit smoking for the first few days, but this is just your body adjusting and getting rid of all the toxins that were settled on your windpipe because of the smoke. This cough is nothing compared to a smokers' cough which is something all smokers suffer from. A smokers' cough is more intense and irritable in comparison to the cough you get when you give up smoking, so this is not a reason for you to hold back your plans of quitting.

Quitting is Expensive

A lot of people believe that they need to spend a ton of money to get over the addiction because they need to enroll themselves in some sort of rehabilitation center or get therapy. Trust me, this is nothing compared to the amount of money you have spent all these years on smoking. On average, people end up spending close to $3,000 annually just on cigarettes. Getting treated permanently will cost you a fraction of that amount.

You Will Fail Anyway

Most smokers make numerous attempts to quit smoking and they still fail. That doesn't mean you give up. You just need to keep trying because smoking is an addiction that is very difficult to overcome and sometimes you may need more than one attempt to quit it. The more times you attempt, the stronger you get so keep trying till you finally succeed.

Conclusion

"The journey of a thousand miles begins with one step." - Lao Tzu

Giving up the addiction of smoking may seem like a long and difficult road to take, but once you have planned the journey, you have already achieved half of what you set out to do. Cigarettes are bad for you and this is something everyone has said multiple times, but unless you decide you want to quit you'll never be able to do it. No-one can make a decision for you and it is something you have to take into your own hands. There are a lot of self-help books out there and handy tips you can use, but the only way you will be able to overcome an addiction is when you put all your effort into it and you don't leave any stone unturned.

Giving yourself leverage is one of the worst things to do because this means you always have the opportunity to go back and smoke. If you want to give up smoking, you have to give it up all at once and not consider cutting down the number of cigarettes that you smoke each day because this will never enable you to quit!

If you want to quit, put out that cigarette and start without turning back ever again!

It is a tough journey but it's something that will help you lead a more fulfilling, healthy and clean life. It's something that will make your loved ones really happy and an achievement you will be extremely proud of.

Begin your journey today and quit smoking like a winner!

"The woods are lovely, dark and deep. But I have promises to keep, and miles to go before I sleep." - Robert Frost

Bonus Material: Earning – An Introduction To

Earning With The Double Your Income Sequence

SECTION 1: THE SECRET OF FORMING MONEY HABITS (AND HOW TO ENFORCE THEM)

You are a collection of your favorite habits.

And, you have a niche set of habits that contribute to the money you can earn and keep, during your average month. Understanding the science behind these habits will help you positively influence the energy you spend on making more money.

A habit is a practice that you have used so often, that it has become an internalized, autonomic

blueprint – a kind of default program for how to execute a specific action.[1]

Habits become damaging when they stop being beneficial, and instead, become uncontrollable, unintentional and contrary to your personal goals. Most individuals carry with them the burden of many bad habits, which inadvertently keeps them from forging ahead and achieving their income goals.

According to Charles Duhigg, the reason why we struggle with habits is that they are as unique as we are. There is no quick-fix formula.

In order to effectively change your habits, you need enlightenment on a better process, and, on your

stuck behavior. Then you can change your *cue-routine-reward* cycle.[2]

> **Cue:** a trigger that puts your brain in automatic mode and chooses your habit
> **Routine:** A physical, mental or emotional set of actions
> **Reward:** What you gain from executing the habit

With fresh ideas and an understanding of how to break bad habit loops, you will adopt powerful new habits that will help you double your income every, single, month.

SECTION 2: HOW TO CREATE NEW MONEY HABITS

New habits are how you will double your income.

This means you need to:

#1: Identify and break bad habits, to free up room for fresh practices
#2: Earnity and consciously adopt new habits, until they become automatic

This guide is not about the first step. If you want to learn how to break bad habits, I suggest reading Charles Duhigg's classic, "The Power of Habit."

What you do need to realize, is that a number of your existing habits need to change, to make room for the ones outlined in this guide. You must become consciously aware of your *cue-routine-reward cycle*, and interrupt it to stay on track.

You can do this effectively by replacing your existing rewards, with your new goal to double your income. To create a new habit, follow this simple process.

- **Identify the bad habit that must be replaced**

  ➢ Waking up at 7 am to be at work at 8 am

- **Identify the harm it's causing**

  ➢ Rushing and feeling harassed and irritated when you get to work

- **Understand and replace the reward from your bad habit**

  ➢ Instead of instant gratification from sleeping late, your mood will be elevated, and your energy levels will be high at work

- **Implement the new habit, motivated by a stronger overall reward**

  ➢ Practice waking up at 5 am, arriving at work at 7:30 and easing into your day, to stimulate the positive mindset required for success

According to modern studies, it takes roughly 66 days before a new behavior becomes automatic.[3]

SECTION 3: THE 14 HABITS THAT WILL DOUBLE YOUR INCOME

Here are the habits you need.

Habit 1: SLEEP (You're Not Doing It Right)

Bill Gates, the co-founder of Microsoft, sleeps for 7 hours every night and reads for 1 hour before bedtime.

With over a third of Americans not getting enough regular sleep, most people vastly underestimate the importance of quality shuteye in their lives.

Over or under-sleeping exposes you to increased risk for chronic conditions, mental distress, stroke and heart disease.[4] According to a 2018 Poll by The National Sleep Foundation, excellent sleepers feel more effective at getting things done the next day.[5]

The first habit you need to adopt is simple – get high quality, regular sleep.

Set a time every evening to go to sleep and stick to it. You should be in bed an hour before, your phone off and all screens far away from you. Read for an hour. Then, go to sleep for 7.

Wake up promptly, 7 hours later. Not a minute more.

Sticking to this new habit promises you stronger immunity, the improved concentration at work and greater emotional stability overall. Consistency will ensure that your circadian rhythms function well, and you never have trouble with restless sleep or with falling asleep.[6]

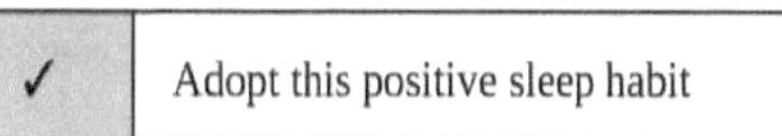

Habit 2: EXERCISE (It's Not Enough, or It's Too Much)

Ex-President Barack Obama works out for 45 minutes a day, six days a week. Thirty minutes or more of aerobic exercise is done daily by 76% of all successful people.[7]

Aerobic exercise is the one consistent habit that will give you the energy you need to succeed. You should run, walk, jog, bike or take a class at the gym. Cardio gets your blood pumping, which is ideal for your brain and boosts your intelligence.[8]

The second habit you need to adopt – find and practice an aerobic exercise, daily.

Now, you need to pick 45 minutes to an hour, every day to get your cardio in. It makes no difference whether you do this in the morning, or late in the evening – as long as it is done every single day.

Consistency is how you will reap these many benefits.

Try to pick something that fits into your life, schedule and likes. You don't have to spend money, you simply have to get active. This means finding an exercise you will enjoy. Some people like boxing classes, others prefer to take a walk around the neighborhood.

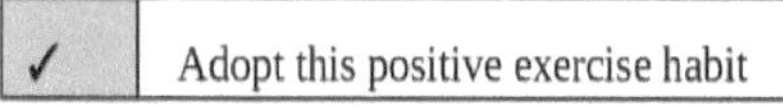

Habit 3: SOCIAL ENERGY (Here's One to Protect)

Oprah Winfrey, talk-show host, and owner of Harpo Studios meditates for 20 minutes every morning, shortly after waking up.

Meditation makes you more in-tune with yourself, how you feel, and how the world around you feels. It's great for focus, increased energy, decreased stress and lifts brain fog.[9]

The people around you have an impact on your energy levels. Successful people surround themselves with positive, go-getters – while the average person is drained by one or more toxic, or negative people in their lives. Social energy must be protected.

The third habit is – to meditate daily on how to optimize your social energy.

According to a Cigna Study, loneliness is at epidemic levels in America.[10] But this is never a good reason to allow anyone a place in your life.
Take a look at your connections and consider if they add, or take energy away from you as you meditate for 20 minutes every morning.

Extroverted, or introverted, you need the right kind of connections in your daily life. If you have energy vampires in your sphere, you must get rid of them to be at your best.

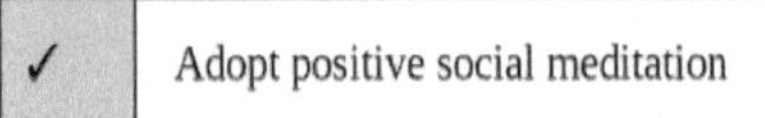

Habit 4: SELF-INVESTMENT (Knowing and Doing)

Albert Einstein believed in constant self-investment through learning, research and application of that newfound knowledge.

The day you stop learning, is the day you stop growing. And personal growth is what takes you towards income acceleration and success. Einstein knew that constant reading was critical to learning, but so was the application of the knowledge learned while reading.

He famously said that too much reading renders the brain lazy. To grow in his field, Einstein continued to study formally until he was 26, then pursued self-study. He was not, as many believe, a naturally talented genius savant – he studied, read and practiced knowledge.[11]

The fourth habit is – invest in your field of knowledge through reading and practice.

If you want to excel like Einstein, shift from consuming entertainment to consuming knowledge. This is easily done by dedicating an hour or more to reading and applying your newly discovered knowledge. Practice what you learn, to see the real difference.[12]

Carve an hour of your day, in the morning or evening to read a book and then realize its lessons. This can be split into 30 minutes of reading, 30 minutes of creating.

 Learn and practice new knowledge

Habit 5: DELEGATION (Focus on The Big Picture)

Richard Branson, Founder of Virgin and hundreds of other companies, is famous for his practice of 'letting go, to grow.' He delegates to focus on the big picture.[13]

Delegation is a habit that most people fail to practice. Instead, they try to do everything themselves and end up burned out, exhausted and depleted.
When you actively practice delegation, you become a talented multitasker, able to orchestrate and design your own career. It is at this point your income will inflate.

The fifth habit is – to practice delegation often and keep your eyes on the big picture.

Your career, or income goals, maybe the big picture for now. Knowing where you want to end up gives you clarity of purpose, and will help you assign what is not important to those around you. This must be done in all aspects of your life that consume your time.

This habit will kick in when someone makes demands on your time. Ask yourself if it contributes to your big picture. If it does not, find a creative way of delegating it to another human being. Make this a habit, and soon you will be surrounded by competent people.[14]

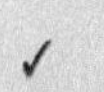 Adopt the habit of delegation

Habit 6: MENTORING (Learning and Teaching)

Marie Forleo is a life coach, philanthropist and entrepreneur, who believes in the power of mentoring and being mentored, to become hugely successful.[15]

In fact, she uses connections to grow her business at every level. With storytelling and the ability to build a community around her lifestyle brand, she was named Oprah's *"thought leader for the next generation."*

Your ability to surround yourself with the right people will be the single most useful habit you can adopt. Most people never actively practice the art of conscious mentoring.

The sixth habit is – to practice attracting network connections that will help you excel!

Who do you know that could teach you something important? Have you ever met someone who you wanted to learn from? Teaching and learning is fundamental to networking, and the basis for all positive relationships, in a corporate environment.[16]

Every day, you should consciously invest more energy in stimulating and improving mentor relationships that will help you grow and succeed as a person in your field. Be ruthlessly selective about your friends and who you spend the most time with.

Allow others to mentor you, and be mentored by you, in a working environment.

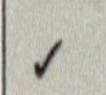 Adopt the habit of mentoring and being mentored

Habit 7: YOUR 96 MINUTES (This is Your Most Valuable Time)

Stephen King is known for his work ethic and ability to produce six good pages of writing every day consistently. He does this by following the same productivity routine daily. [17]

You need to have the discipline and consistency required, to do something for your direct productivity benefit, for 96 minutes a day. Why 96 minutes?

Science says that everyone has 96 highly productive minutes every day, a time window when you have the most energy and are at your best. If you harness this power and use it for your ultimate goal of earning more money, it shifts from possible, to probable.[18]

The seventh habit is – Spend 96 minutes a day working on your main career goal.

Discover when your 96 minutes kicks in. It might be just after waking up. It might be late at night when everyone else is sleeping. Find your window and use it.

Spend those 96 minutes focused exclusively on your main career goal. If that is to get a promotion, this is when you will plan and execute a strategy. If it is to launch a website, this is when you will put in the work.

 Adopt the 96-minute habit

Habit 8: INNOVATION (Get to The Core of Things)

Elon Musk, the founder of PayPal, SpaceX and Tesla, is a known innovator and practices the Richard Feynman technique mixed with first principles, to stay creative. [19]

The underlying concept of this technique is to not try and remember, but to understand – because when you do, you automatically remember. It's a way to entertain new ideas and be creative in a way that promotes productivity.

Knowledge to Elon, is about understanding the fundamental principles of a thing, to know the trunk and branches before diving headlong into the details, or the leaves of an idea.

The eighth habit is – when learning something new, to understand its core first.

Applying this to your career will make you a forward-thinking innovator. For example, if you are a psychologist, you would benefit from learning more about neuroscience, because it is at the core of your field. Competency is all about strong, unshakable fundamentals.[20]

Spend 30 minutes every day learning something that reinforces how you innovate in your chosen field. Soon you will be questioning, brainstorming and seeing patterns that may amount to improvements you can implement.

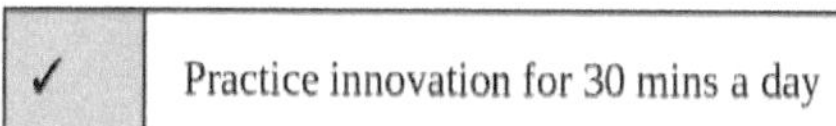

Habit 9: THE WIN-WIN (Mutually Beneficial Relationships)

Stephen Covey, author of the smash hit "The 7 Habits of Highly Effective People" advocated the importance of win-win relationships.

According to Covey, most people approach life with a scarcity mindset, as opposed to an abundance mindset. Because of this, social interactions become unbalanced.[21]

There are several types of human interaction, win-lose, lose-lose, lose-win – but none are as powerful or effective as the win-win. When you practice win-win interactions, your engagements are mutually beneficial, and people will enjoy working with you.

The ninth habit is – to practice win-win human interactions in your daily life.

When you do, you will find that people flock to you, because they see the benefits of doing business with you. When everyone benefits, you can succeed together.

This habit will cue when someone asks you for something. This should be your trigger to think about how you can make the interaction a win-win scenario. Covey says, to take consideration and courage into account, and to be creative in your problem-solving.

As you create win-win results, your influence will grow in your field. Remember that there is enough success around for everyone, and you can create it for them!

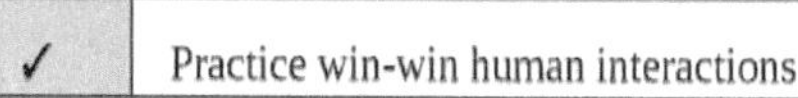

Habit 10: SPEAK UP (Know and Communicate Your Value)

Tyra Banks, ex-supermodel, TV producer and personality, based her career success on the ability to speak up, negotiate and get what she desires most.

She made a habit of speaking clearly, frankly and openly about her value with the people around her. Too often, we get stuck in the habit of remaining passive, and silent about our worth. Promotions and opportunities will pass you by because you failed to speak up.

The tenth habit is – to speak up when necessary about your value as an employee.

Tyra explains, that it is a shift from an 'I need' to an 'I deserve' mindset. Instead of explaining to your employer why you need a raise, you should explain why you deserve one. This is easily done by focusing on your value – or how you positively contribute to the company.[22]

This is another habit that will cue when you identify opportunities or feel that you deserve a promotion at your job. In meetings, be open about your contributions to the success of projects or initiatives. Speak up about how you, as a person, make things better.

Getting into the habit of communicating your worth to people around you, positions you for rapid advancement. If you cannot see and communicate your value, the higher-ups will not see it either. Be persistent. Have a clear voice. And do not get lost in the crowd.

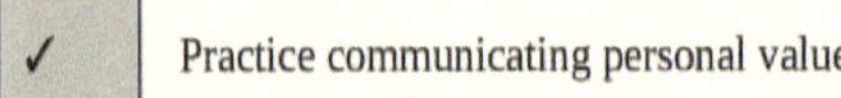

Habit 11: PAY YOURSELF FIRST (This is Ground-breaking Advice)

George Clason was the author who wrote the classic 'The Richest Man in Babylon' and taught people to pay themselves first, in order to gain real wealth.[23]

Imagine if, since you had started working at age 21, you had put away 10% of every paycheck. This is what it means to pay yourself first. Money saved and kept earns compound interest and grows exponentially over long periods of time.

People that want to be wealthy use this strategy to move from employed earning to investing. Investing money is how you break out of your income bracket altogether.

The eleventh habit is – to put 10% of every paycheck aside to grow your wealth.

It might seem like very little at first, but 5 years of putting away just $100.00, frees up $6000.00 for investment. It gives you options to supplement your salary as you age.

To start the habit, every time you are paid – immediately take 10% of that total amount and put it in a separate account. You cannot touch this money. It is there simply to exist and earn you money from long-term growth.

The pay yourself first habit will help you clear away your debt, and get you investing at a young age. Get into this habit early, and you will benefit from time itself.

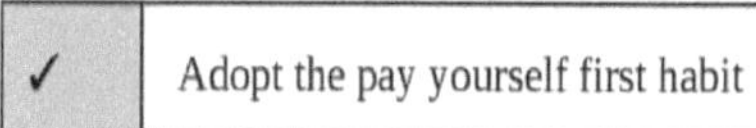

Habit 12: SIDE HUSTLE (Spend Your Time for Returns)

Rob Kalin never meant Etsy.com to be such a smash success. Initially, it was simply his side hustle, born from a desire to make wood-encased computers. [24]

Rob Kalin is a furniture designer who started Etsy as a place to sell his wares. It was a side hustle, an increasingly common play among Millennials. Some 61% of Millennials work on their side hustles once a week or more.[25]

This is usually a job that earns them money beyond their 9-5, or a personal project with income potential that they are developing. What is your side hustle?

The twelfth habit is – work on your side hustle twice a week.

On Mondays and Thursdays, or Tuesdays and Fridays you should dedicate a couple of hours to your side hustle. This is a second business, born from your creative or analytical talents that may become a solid earner for you down the line.

Scheduling in time to develop your secondary projects is important for personal growth, and increasing your income. Many Millennials discover that once their side businesses reach a certain level, they can either sell them or commit fulltime to their passions.

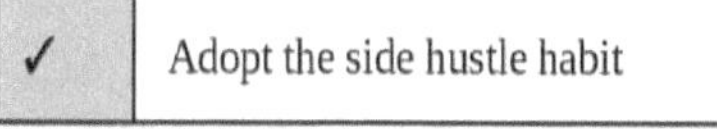

Habit 13: SUNDAY REVIEW (3 Hours to Financial Freedom!)

Suze Orman, a personal finance expert and personality, is known for teaching people to pick just one thing about their finances to work on, at a time. [26]

She called it the 'one and done' method, and it simplifies the huge challenge of getting hold of your financial situation. Many people find their finances overwhelming, and so never take proactive steps towards understanding and controlling them.

The thirteenth habit is – to spend 3 hours every Sunday focusing on one financial problem.

You might need to save, or clear debt, or better understand your expenses and how to curb them. Whatever you need, you will tackle it during a designated time, every Sunday.

When you practice the habit of reviewing your finances regularly, to better understand and control them, you will change your life.

Make sure that you pick only one simple thing at a time so that you can properly digest and institute changes as necessary. Spend the time learning and streamlining for your ultimate benefit, as a responsible financial planner.

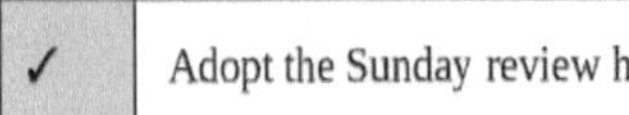

Habit 14: MINIMALISM (Know How to Spend)

Steve Jobs, Founder of Apple, was a noted minimalist and wore the same black turtleneck every day for many, many years.

Popularized by Silicon Valley, minimalism reduces decision-fatigue, a common problem in today's overcrowded, ultra-informed society. With so much information and choice out there, it is no wonder you struggle to make good decisions for yourself. [27]

The theory goes that you can only make so many strong decisions in a day. The minimalist habit, allows you to dedicate those decisions to things that matter, like spending for value.

The fourteenth habit is – to spend with minimalism in mind.

Consumer culture is not for the truly rich. Instead, these individuals spend more money on a single item of quality, than repeated spending on numerous low-quality items.

Get into the habit of spending money on quality items, instead of cheaper items that will wear and degrade. This will free up your time as you make fewer wardrobe decisions. Instead of spending your creative energy there, you will spend it at work, where it matters most.

Less items of higher quality will simplify and improve your life.

<table>
<tr><td>✓</td><td>Adopt the spending for value habit</td></tr>
</table>

SECTION 4: THE GOLDEN RULE OF SUCCESS SEQUENCING

Your habits determine your behavior, but one thing is more important.

Focus.

Your attention is a form of currency that will either enrich or impoverish your life. That is why they call it 'paying attention.' Focus is the literal gateway to learning, reasoning, decision-making, problem-solving and perception.[28]

That is why consistent focus on your habits is the golden rule of success.

None of the people you have read about in this guide could have succeeded without an all-encompassing focus on their daily habits. Every individual here keeps a rigorous, personalized schedule that optimizes these habits.

Success, like your daily habits, is incredibly personal. Only you can decide when you have achieved a high enough level of success. And your habits are the stepping stones!

If you want to double your income, nothing is keeping you from it, but your habits. When you remove the bad and replace it with these powerful income-generating habits, you will immediately experience rapid change that will reshape your life.

That is why your primary focus must be a habitual practice, according to a personalized schedule. Without it, expect to fall back into bad patterns of behavior.

SECTION 5: THESE HABITS WILL MATTER MOST!

According to a study from Northwestern University, a domino effect happens when you adopt one lasting good habit.[29]

In other words, exercising every day will encourage positive eating habits. In turn, this may spread to you getting better quality sleep and performing better at work. Management of these small, seemingly insignificant habits starts with internalizing just one.

I want you to pick a habit from this list to act as your linchpin habit.

Then I want you to dedicate the next 66 days to internalizing that habit, and when you feel capable, adopt more from this list.

Even if you struggle to adopt more of these habits, I want you to commit to just the one. At no point over the next 66 days will you, at any point, stop practicing that habit.

The first couple in this list have the most impact. They directly affect your daily performance. This is how you will naturally double your income in the short term.

Consider the domino effect active in you right now. But it is focused on negative habits. Switch to replacing them with positive habits, and you will soar!

The habits that matter most are the ones you learn to keep. Make them part of who you are, and soon you will leap an income bracket.

SECTION 6: WILLPOWER OR WONTPOWER: YOU DECIDE

The number 1 barrier to change is a mysterious thing called 'willpower.'

Those who have it are strong. Those who lack willpower are weak.

That is what we are taught to believe in our modern society. Your ability to resist short-term temptations is chalked up to your measure of willpower.

But you are never told what it is, or how to get it. How is it meant to take over, when you have no idea how it works?

Now I am going to lift the veil.

Willpower is little more than self-control. It is the conscious act of choosing what is right, over what is easy. It is picking cognition, over emotion. It is discipline.[30]

Willpower is a *habit*.

Right now, you habitually give in to your desires. What you need to do is replace this with your long-term plan for success. Say no to instant gratification!

Practice consciously choosing to focus on what is most important, every day.

If you don't want to exercise, use your willpower. Emotions drive your thoughts. Replace them with conscious thoughts that are more beneficial. You must exercise, to feel good today, tomorrow, this week. You must exercise to earn more and be better.

Practice willpower as a habit, and soon it will take over.

SECTION 7: REGAINING YOUR FAITH IN FREE WILL

'But I have so much to do.'
'I'll begin after my major project is over.'
'I'll just let this week pass, and I'll be ready.'

It is human nature to wait for the ideal time to change. You might have bought this guide with the intent to adopt these habits 'at some point.'

This is because you have lost faith in free will. Free will is your ability to choose between different courses of action, unimpeded. Now, life is all about impediments, but that does not mean you cannot choose to be better. You can.

We are all made up of a unique blend of strengths, weaknesses, circumstances and perceptions. Your free will must be exercised in accordance with your make-up, within your unique context, under your special circumstances.

The price of freedom is struggling.

The price of earning more is learning to be better.[31]

Then being better – every day!
If you cannot be better consistently, hope is lost.
In this way, free will gives you the opportunity to be whoever you want, as long as you are willing to go through the wringer to get there. It will be hard! If it were easy, everyone would be successful and living these rare lives.

My advice to be something is to practice.
Start and start *today*.

Check Out Our Other AMAZING Titles:

1. *Resolving Anxiety and Panic Attacks*

A Guide to Overcoming Severe Anxiety, Controlling Panic Attacks and Reclaiming Your Life Again

Worldwide, one in six people is affected by a mental health disorder. So you are not alone in this (Ritchie & Roser, 2019). There is a difference between clinical anxiety and everyday anxiety. Everyday anxiety is normal and in often cases, it is necessary, while chronic anxiety will leave you functionally impaired. This book will not only inform you about anxiety and panic attacks but also introduce you to various methods and techniques that aid in getting rid of anxiety. It is a perfect package if you want to make long-lasting, meaningful changes in your life in a way that gets rid of anxiety. Knowledge is power, so gaining information about anxiety and panic attacks already puts you in the lead against them.

In the first chapter, we'll start with the basic knowledge of panic attacks and anxiety. The symptoms of both are pretty much the same, but there are some major differences as well. Knowing their difference and similarities can help you clearly understand your condition. Some basic ways of coping with them are also explained alongside their symptoms.

After gaining knowledge about anxiety and panic attacks in the first section, you will seek answers and ways to overcome them. The second chapter goes more in detail about the physical effects of anxiety. There are some types of anxiety which are also talked briefly about in the chapter. There are also therapies and treatments that are used to overcome and control anxiety. Their details are discussed in the chapter from where you can figure out what sort of treatment will suit you better. Some other ways of coping with anxiety are also discussed and they will surely prove beneficial to the reader.

The third chapter will make you aware of how interrelated physical and mental healths are. There are also details on how to improve one's physical health to influence a person's anxiety positively. You will also learn how important practicing well-being is. If you are to ignore physical health, it will cause problems for your mental health as well.

The fourth chapter will delve deep into mindfulness and its vast benefits. Mindfulness is a very powerful tool we have but don't know how to use. It can be practiced through meditation techniques, etc. It makes us see things more clearly than ever before. Practicing Mindfulness will arm you against any anxiety and panic attacks. In this chapter, it is explained in detail what it means and what are its advantages.

In the fifth chapter, we will learn about meditation and how can it help manage anxiety. We first start off by knowing what it is. You also have got to know its benefits and various techniques from which one can pick according to their choice. We will also learn the accurate posture you should have during meditation. We will learn how mediation reinforces our brain to stave off anxiety and panic attacks. It is a long road but a successful one for sure. Besides helping us out with anxiety and panic disorder, meditation has numerous other benefits for our body and mind.

The sixth chapter will explore the meaning behind self-love and its importance in fighting anxiety. Our battle with anxiety has to start from a positive ground. We first have to be fully comfortable and respectful towards ourselves. You will also find out how lack of self-love can actually breed anxiety.

Opening about anxiety is not an easy task but could be very helpful against anxiety. How to go about the whole process is talked about in detail in the seventh chapter. You will also learn how to evaluate your therapist and choose the right one. In this chapter, there are also guidelines for people who have just recently become aware of their anxiety and now they want to seek help. It will give them knowledge about things to consider when talking to someone about mental health, what you should accept and be prepared for. There is also information about talk therapy there.

In the eighth chapter, we address the misunderstanding about anxiety. Despite affecting so many people, it remains a different experience for all of them. There are also common mistakes pointed out in that chapter which we'll go into detail the mistakes that make our anxiety worse.

The ninth chapter is about where we talk about putting our foot down and start to incorporate practices into our life which will help you get rid of anxiety and panic attacks. We will learn how to manage our responses. It is basically a comprehensive listing of all the things you should be avoiding or adapting to lead a healthy lifestyle free of anxiety.

*Want to read more? Purchase our book on **Anxiety and Panic Attacks** today!*

2. *Cognitive Behavioral Therapy*

How CBT Can Be Used to Rewire Your Brain, Stop Anxiety, and Overcome Depression

Cognitive stems from cognition, which encapsulates the idea of how we learn and the knowledge that we carry. The things you learn are part of your cognition, and what you do with that information is included in that category as well. Cognition includes a wide list of information that you might not fully realize.

Behavior is what we do. It is how we act. The things that you choose to say to other people are all about your behavior. How you react to what others have to say will exhibit your behavior as well. Your behavior is all about your mind interacting with your body and how that interacts with the people and other things that surround you.

Therapy is any form of help, usually from a trained professional, to help improve on whatever the therapy is specified for. You might get physical therapy to help regain strength in your knee after having a serious surgery. You can also get therapy to help overcome an alcohol or drug addiction.

Throughout this book, we're going to give you the basis you need to start understanding cognitive behavioral therapy. The three together—cognitive, behavioral, therapy—all make up CBT, which is a method that is going to directly help you overcome the mental illness that you are hoping to treat.

Therapy can be expensive, and even if you do have the means to go through with this process, you might struggle to find the right therapist. Sometimes, you might live in an area where there is only one therapist within a close distance, but you don't have a vibe with them that you find to be helpful. You might also find that you are desperate for help and that you want a therapist, but insurance coverage isn't always good for this.

By reading this book, you'll be able to find the tools you need to help with overcoming your most challenging thoughts. We are going to take you through the steps to identify the root issues and come up with specific methods to get you through.

*Want to read more? Purchase our book on **Cognitive Behavioral Therapy** today!*

3. *Effective Guide On How to Sleep Well Everyday*

The Easy Method For Better Sleep, Insomnia And Chronic Sleep Problems

"A well spent day brings happy sleep." — Leonardo da Vinci

Are you experiencing the worst restless feeling? Has your doctor diagnosed you with insomnia, restlessness, sleeplessness? When the whole world around you seems to be in peaceful deep slumber, you are the one who is restless. No matter what term is used to describe it, the fact is that it is you who is actually going through insomnia, and nothing could feel worse than that.

So you drag yourself from bed in the morning feeling as earth, with its entire lock stock and barrel, has decided to perch on your head for the day. Yet you go through the motions of the day, though you barely manage to make it through the hours. By the early night, you fall on to bed hoping this night will be different because you're dead tired and nothing will keep you from sleeping like a log. It's 2.00 a.m. now, dawn is breaking through and there you are, still wide awake and ready to scream to the world because no matter how tired you are or how hard you have tried, you simply can't get to sleep.

While there are proven facts and evidence of the devastating effects of sleeping less, the investigations are still on to establish the exact nature of effects resulting from too much sleep. Some researchers argue that people who sleep much longer than necessarily have a higher death rate. Physical and mental conditions such as depression or socioeconomic status can also lead to excessive sleep. There are other researchers who argue that the human body will naturally restrain it from sleeping more hours than really necessary. However, with research still underway for concrete evidence of the effects of over sleeping the best path you can choose is to adopt a sleeping pattern somewhere in the middle. According to the National Sleep Foundation, this middle range falls between seven and eight hours of sleep during the night. Despite these statistics, the best way to ensure you receive sufficient sleeping time is to let your own body act as your guide. You can always sleep a little extra if you feel exhausted or sleep a little less than usual if you feel you are oversleeping.

Dangers of Sleep deprivation.

Though sleep is something the average human being takes for granted, it is also one of the greatest mysteries in life. Just like we still don't have all the answers to the quantum field or gravity, researchers are still exploring the reasons behind the 'whats' and 'whys' of sleep. However, one fact unchallenged about sleep is that a proper sleep is paramount for maintaining good health. The general guideline regarding the optimal amount of sleep for an adult range from six to eight hours! If you carry on with too little or too much of this general guideline you are exposing yourself to the risk of adverse health effects.

Though sleep is something that comes naturally to many people, the problems of sleep deprivation have today become a pressing problem with more and more people succumbing to chronic sleeping disorders. Unfortunately, a great number of these people do not even realize that lack of sleep or sleep deprivation is at the root of their manifold problems in life. Scientific research also points out that lack of sleep on a continuous scale can lead to severe repercussions on your health.

If you have been experiencing impaired sleep patterns for a longer period, you also face the risk of:

- Severely impairing your immunity strength

- Promoting the risk of tumor growth, as it has been scientifically established that a tumor can grow at least two to three times faster among animals subjected to severe sleeping dysfunctions within a laboratory setting.

- Creating a pre-diabetic condition in the body. Insomnia creates hunger, making you want to eat even when you have already had a meal. This situation can lead to problems of obesity in turn.

- Critically impairing memory. How many times during the day have you found it difficult to remember even the most mundane and repetitive events when you have had no more than 4 – 5 hours of sleep? Even a single night of impaired sleep plays havoc with our memory faculties, just think what it can do to your brain if you consistently lose sleep.

- Ruining your performance level both physically and mentally as your problem-solving abilities will not be working in peak order.

- Stomach ulcers

- Constipation, hemorrhoids

- Heart diseases

- Depression, lethargy and other mood disorders

- Daytime drowsiness

- Irritability

- Low energy

- Low mental clarity

- Reaction time slows down

- Lower productivity

- More accidents and mistakes

- Lower levels of growth hormone and testosterone

The growth hormone in the body which is vital for maintaining our looks, energy, and skin texture is produced by the pituitary gland. The specialty of this hormone production procedure is that it is only produced during the times of deep slumber or during intense workout sessions. In the absence of normal production of the growth hormone, our bodies will start on a premature aging process. According to research, people suffering from chronic insomnia are three times more susceptible to contract fatal diseases. When you lose sleep overnight, you cannot make up for it by sleeping more the next day. A night's lost sleep will be lost forever. More alarmingly if you continue to lose sleep regularly, they will create a cumulative negative effect that will disrupt your general health. All in all, sleeping deficiencies can effectively make your life miserable, as you already know.

How Much Sleep Do I Really Need?

This is a question that remains a mystery just like the questions of why and what makes us want to sleep. In response to a question of how many hours of sleep do we really need, an expert has answered that it is actually lot less than what we have been taught. On the other hand, though a good night's sleep is vital for good health, overdoing the sleeping can be equally bad for us. But if you sleep less and continue this for too long, the result will be confusion between body and brain signals, resulting in muddled thoughts, lethargic feelings, and overall lassitude. So, the question remains, how many hours of sleep do we really need? Is it essential to sleep the prescribed number of eight hours a day or is catching up a good sleep on a five to six-hour basis enough?

The eight hours of sleep theory is increasingly becoming unpractical in this fast-paced lifestyle. Actually, the recommendation of eight hours of sleep arises based on the idea that our ancestors had their beauty sleep between 8-9 hours in the past. In today's context, this concept is regarded more or less as a myth. In a study conducted by the Sleep Research Center, youngsters within the age group of 8 to 17 generally sleep for about nine hours during the night. However, in the case of adults, this theory is not applicable as a majority of them are sleepless and many of them thrive after a solid sleep varying between 5-7 hours.

A research conducted by the National Institute of Health has established that people who sleep soundly for nine hours a day or more are actually two times more vulnerable than those who sleep less in developing Parkinson's disease. A study report released by the Diabetes Care states that people claiming to sleep less than five hours or more than nine hours daily are the ones with the highest risk of attracting diabetes. In contrast, a large number of contemporary studies prove that people with sleeping patterns that do not exceed or fall beyond seven hours daily possess the highest survival rate. The persons who experience sleeping disorders and sleep less than 4.5 hours have the worst survival rate.

When ascertaining the correct number of hours you should sleep, the fact is that there is no magic number of hours. It will depend on a person to person basis as well as factors like age, activity, and performance level. For example, smaller children and teenagers require more sleep compared to adults. Your personal requirements will not be the same as your friend or colleague who is of the same age and gender as you. Because your sleep needs are unique and individual. According to the National Sleep Foundation, the difference of sleep requirements between two people of the same age, gender, and activity level is due to their basal sleep needs and sleep debt.

Your basal sleep need is the number of hours of sleep you typically need to engage in optimal performance levels. The sleep debt comprises of the accumulated number of hours of sleep you have lost as a result of poor sleeping habits, a recent sickness, social demands, environmental factors, etc. A healthy adult generally possesses a basal sleep need between seven and eight hours each night. If you have experienced sleeping difficulties and as a result accumulated a sleep debt you will find that your performance level is not up to its usual standard, even if you wake up after seven or eight hours of restful sleep. The symptoms will be most apparent during the times the circadian rhythm naturally alters like during mid-afternoon or overnight. One of the ways of easing out of an accumulated sleep debt situation is to get a few extra hours of sleep for a couple of nights until you regain your natural sleeping rhythm and vitality during the day.

Understand what Kind of a Sleeper Are You?

Sleep, dear reader, is the precious restorative that rights so many physical and mental wrongs. The elixir that transforms life and puts a spring in your step, a smile on your face, and the feeling that you can take care of everything that comes your way is sleep. Undervalued, ignored, and forgotten until you wake up to the realization that it's one of the essential foundations of daily wellbeing.

So what kind of a sleeper are you? There are many studies and descriptions of how we sleep but the common consensus settles for the following five simple categories:

1. Lively, healthy early risers!

These happy individuals usually get the sleep they need and rarely feel exhausted or fatigued. They are typically younger than the other groups, usually married or with a long-term partner, working full-time and definitely a morning person with no serious medical conditions.

2. Relaxed and retired seniors.

This is the oldest group in the survey with half of the sample being 65 or older. They sleep the most with an average of 7.3 hours per night compared to 6.8 across all groups. Sleep disorders are rare even though there is a significant proportion with at least one medical disorder.

3. Dozing drones.

These busy people are usually married/partnered and employed but they often work much longer than forty hours a week. Frequently working up to the hour when they go to bed, they get up early so they're always short of sleep and struggle to keep up with the daily pressures of life. Statistically, they'll feel tired or fatigued at least three days a week.

4. Galley slaves.

This group works the longest hours and often suffers from weight problems as well as an unhealthy reliance on caffeine to get through the day. Shift workers often fall into this group and there is also a marked tendency to be a night owl or evening person. They get the least amount of sleep and are more likely to take naps yet, surprisingly, this group often believes that, despite the state of their health, they are getting enough sleep.

5. Insomniacs.

Here is the largest proportion of night people and many of them quite rightly believe they have a sleep problem. About half of this group feel they get less sleep than they need and the same proportion admits to feeling tired, fatigued and lacking energy most of the time.

So, which of the five groups do you think you fit into?

If you're a happy member of Group One, your sleep should by definition be absolutely fine. Don't worry. We've got some really good ideas to share with you to keep you right on track and we'll even add some special extra features to your nightly rest routine to maximize the experience. If you're not in this group, our aim is to help you become a full-time member of the healthy, happy sleepers' association! Membership is for life.

Group Three represents too many tired, irritable, and generally inefficient individuals whose quality of life is impaired because they're too tired too often. Their work suffers because they rarely have sufficient rest to successfully assimilate the day's events. Their home life is degraded because work intrudes too often and they're just too tired to enjoy the pleasures and comfort of a life away from work. Feeling tired becomes their default position and they know they need to do something to give their minds and bodies the rest they deserve. Individuals in this group frequently suffer from long- term mental, physical and emotional stress.

The fourth group is rightly described as the night owls. They work the longest hours and, as we noted above, they typically work shifts. The health problems associated with this group include a marked tendency towards obesity as well as a range of inflammatory diseases. Despite the fact that these people rarely look or feel well, they seem to ignore the evidence and usually claim to get enough sleep, relying on sugary energy drinks and caffeine to keep them awake during waking hours. They take naps because their bodies can't function without additional sleep during the day. An objective analysis of their health would typically reveal a range of health and wellbeing issues.

Insomniacs are the dominant members of Group Five, people who don't get enough sleep, can't get to sleep, and who know they have a problem. Unfortunately, many insomniacs end up taking prescription medication to deal with their symptoms and we have to question the benefits of this solution in light of the many unpleasant side effects associated with long-term sleeping pill dependency. For insomniacs, life is a constant struggle because of the accumulative effects of long-term sleep deprivation.

Health issues abound, depression becomes a major risk, their ability to function normally is often impaired, and they lose sight of their potential to deal successfully with life's daily challenges. They sometimes refer to their condition as living in a nightmare world where they are constantly exhausted and simply cannot function. It's completely understandable that a doctor would prescribe sleeping drugs because the dangers of sleep deprivation can be acute.

Before we begin to examine the practicalities of sleep, we need to know how much sleep is appropriate for each of us as individuals. It's not surprising that different age groups have different sleep requirements.

For example, very young children and infants can sleep in total for around 14 - 15 hours a day. And if you've got teenagers, you might have guessed that adolescents usually need more sleep than adults. Teens can easily sleep between 8.5 to 9.5 hours a night.

It's widely understood that during the first trimester, pregnant women often find they need a lot more sleep than usual. The fact is that if you feel tired during the day, find yourself yawning or taking a nap, you're short on sleep. And this is the time for you to do something practical, realistic, and effective to take care of the problem.

There are many myths surrounding the condition known as OAS or Obstructive Sleep Apnea. It's estimated that around 18 million Americans suffer from the condition but the numbers could be much higher because many people don't report the condition to their doctors. This condition is far more than just loud snoring, although snoring can be a sign of sleep apnea.

People with this condition skip breathing 400 times during the night. The delay in breathing can last from ten to thirty seconds and is then followed by a loud snore as breathing suddenly resumes. The normal sleep cycle is interrupted and this can leave sufferers feeling tired and exhausted during the day. It is a serious condition, especially since it can lead to accidents at work, problems when driving, as well as increasing the risk of heart attacks and strokes. It can affect people of all ages, including children, but tends to affect people more after the age of forty.

Weight also plays a part and there is evidence that shedding excess pounds can improve the condition. Despite all the advice and overwhelming evidence, there are still surprising numbers of sleep apnea sufferers who continue to smoke. Smoking is a perfect way to increase the severity and risks of this debilitating condition.

If you've already trimmed your weight, quit smoking and tried sleeping on your side but still suffer from the condition, you need to see your doctor. There are many treatments available including a special mask that delivers constant air flow to keep the breathing passage open. Lifestyle choices can clearly make a positive difference, too.

Your body, your brain, your mind and your emotional functioning all rely on sufficient sleep to operate efficiently. If you don't get enough sleep, everything suffers. Research suggests that it's much harder than you might imagine to adapt having less sleep than your body needs. The sleep deficit has to be repaid at some point or we'll experience increasingly severe problems.

Simple techniques of preparing for bed

1. Try to get to bed early. The recharging of the body's adrenal system usually takes place between 11p.m. and 1a.m. in the morning. The gallbladder uses the same time to release the toxin build up in the body. If you happen to be awake when both these functions are taking place within your body, there is the possibility of the toxin backing up to the liver which can endanger your health very badly. Sleeping late are byproducts of modern living styles. However, the human body was created in synchronization of nature and its activities. That is why before the advent of electricity people used to go to bed just after sundown and wake up with sunrise.

2. Don't alter your bedtimes haphazardly. Try to stick to a pattern where you go to bed and wake up at the same time. This should be done even on weekends. The continuous pattern will help your body to fit into a rhythm.

3. Maintain a soothing bedtime routine. This can change from person to person. You can use deep breathing exercises, meditation, use of aromatherapy, a gentle relaxing massage given by your partner,

or even going through a complete and relaxing skin care routine. The secret is to get into a rhythm which makes you comfortable, relaxed, and ready for bed. Repeating it every day will help in easing out the tensions of the day.

4. Refrain from taking any heavy fluids two hours before bed time. This habit will minimize the number of times you need to visit the bathroom in the middle of the night. You should also make a habit of going to the bathroom just before you get into bed, so that you will not get the urge during night time.

5. Eat a meal enriched with proteins several hours before your bed time. The protein will enhance the production of L-tryptophan which is essential for the production of serotonin and melatonin. Follow up your meal with some fruit to help the tryptophan to cross easily across the blood brain barrier.

6. Refrain from taking any snacks while in bed or just before bed and reduce the level of sugar and grains in your dinner time as it will raise the blood sugar level, delaying sleep. When the body starts metabolizing these elements and the blood sugar level start dropping you will find yourself suddenly awake and unable to go back to sleep.

7. A hot bath before bed is found to be very soothing. When the body temperature is stimulated to a raised level during late evening by the time you get into bed, it will be ready to drop, signaling slumber time to your brain.

8. Stop your work and put them away ideally one to two hours before bed. The interval between work and bedtime should be used for unwinding from the pressure and tension of work. It is essential that you approach your bed with a calm mind instead of being hyped up about some matter.

9. If you prefer reading, a novel with an uplifting story instead of a stimulating one like suspense or mystery is recommended. Or the suspense will keep you up half the night awake trying to visualize the end to the mystery!

A Few Lifestyle Suggestions to Make You Sleep Better

Don't take medications and drugs unless it is absolutely necessary for your health and wellbeing. A majority of prescribed and over the counter drugs can cause changes in your sleeping patterns.

Avoid drinks with alcohol or caffeine. Caffeine takes longer to metabolize in the body so that your body will experience its effects much longer after consumption. That is why even the cup of coffee you had in the evening will keep you awake during the night. Some of the medications and drugs in the market also contain caffeine which account for their capacity to generate sleeping irregularities. Though alcohol can make you feel drowsy the effect is very much short lived. Once the feeling goes away, you will find that sleep is eluding you for many hours and even the sleep that you finally reach will not take you to deep slumber after alcohol. In the absence of deep sleep, your body will not be able to perform its usual healing and regeneration process is vital for lasting healthiness.

Engage in regular exercise activities. If you are contained in an 8-hour office job, you should make sure that your body receives plenty of exercise which can dramatically increase your sleep health. The best time to exercise is, however, not closer to your bedtime but in the morning.

Keep away from sensitive food types that will keep you awake at night like sugar, pasteurized dairy foods, and grains. These foods can result in congestion, leading to gastric disorders.

The sleep apnea risk is enhanced amongst people with weight issues. If you think you have gained a few extra pounds and during this time you have also experienced sleeping trouble focus on losing the extra weight as a priority. The sleeping issue will correct automatically.

If your body is going through a hormone upheaval like during menopausal or premenopausal time, seek advice from your family physician, as this time can lead to sleeping difficulties.

*Want to read more? Purchase our book on **Effective Guide On How to Sleep***